Nursing Aid

Artificial Kidney Dialysis Unit and Operation Theater Techniques

Nursing Aid

Artificial Kidney Dialysis Unit and Operation Theater Techniques

Cecilia Correia

Ex-Nursing Tutor
Cardinal Gracious Memorial Hospital
Vasai, Maharashtra

CBS Publishers & Distributors Pvt Ltd

New Delhi • Bengaluru • Chennai • Kochi • Kolkata • Mumbai
Bhopal • Bhubaneswar • Hyderabad • Jharkhand • Nagpur • Patna
• Pune • Uttarakhand • Dhaka (Bangladesh) • Kathmandu (Nepal)

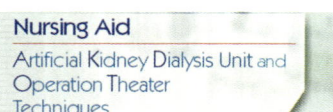

Nursing Aid
Artificial Kidney Dialysis Unit and Operation Theater Techniques

ISBN: 978-81-239-2848-7

Copyright © Author and Publisher

First Edition: 2016
Reprint: 2020

Published by Satish Kumar Jain and Produced by Varun Jain for

CBS Publishers & Distributors Pvt Ltd

4819/XI Prahlad Street, 24 Ansari Road, Daryaganj, New Delhi 110 002, India.
Ph: 23289259, 23266861, 23266867   Fax: 011-23243014   Website: www.cbspd.com
e-mail: delhi@cbspd.com; cbspubs@airtelmail.in.
Corporate Office: 204 FIE, Industrial Area, Patparganj, Delhi 110 092
Ph: 4934 4934   Fax: 4934 4935   e-mail: publishing@cbspd.com; publicity@cbspd.com

Branches

- **Bengaluru:** Seema House 2975, 17th Cross, K.R. Road, Banasankari 2nd Stage, Bengaluru 560 070, Karnataka
  Ph: +91-80-26771678/79   Fax: +91-80-26771680   e-mail: bangalore@cbspd.com
- **Chennai:** 7, Subbaraya Street, Shenoy Nagar, Chennai 600 030, Tamil Nadu
  Ph: +91-44-26260666, 26208620   Fax: +91-44-42032115   e-mail: chennai@cbspd.com
- **Kochi:** 42/1325, 1326, Power House Road, Opp KSEB Power House, Ernakulam 682 018, Kochi, Kerala
  Ph: +91-484-4059061-65   Fax: +91-484-4059065   e-mail: kochi@cbspd.com
- **Kolkata:** No. 6/B, Ground Floor, Rameswar Shaw Road, Kolkata-700014 (West Bengal), India
  Ph: +91-33-2289-1126, 2289-1127, 2289-1128   e-mail: kolkata@cbspd.com
- **Mumbai:** 83-C, Dr E Moses Road, Worli, Mumbai-400018, Maharashtra
  Ph: +91-22-24902340/41   Fax: +91-22-24902342   e-mail: mumbai@cbspd.com

Representatives

• Bhopal	0-8319310552	• Bhubaneswar	0-9911037372	• Hyderabad	0-9885175004
• Jharkhand	0-9811541605	• Nagpur	0-9421945513	• Patna	0-9334159340
• Pune	0-9623451994	• Uttarakhand	0-9716462459	• Dhaka	01912-003485
• Kathmandu (Nepal)	977-9818742655				

Printed at HT Media Ltd., Greater Noida, UP, India

to

my best friend Sheelu
who is a medical person and has played multidimensional roles in
the field of education, managing an educational institution on her own.
May her dedication and commitment be an example and inspiration,
radiating peace to all those who read this book.

to love without condition, to talk without intention, to give without reason
and to care without expectation, is the heart of true relation.
What we do for us dies with us, what we do for others lives into immortality

Preface

First time in my nursing career when I visited the AKD (artificial kidney dialysis) unit, I was back to my place feeling hopeless. I was just silent and feeling uneasy. I just looked at God and this just came out of my lips, Oh God, why this suffering. I saw very young to elderly, rich to very poor, and patients of all religions and casts in the unit under dialysis. There were just plain faces with no expressions of joy, looking at you with hope, "will I live long enough after this dialysis? Is there any other way without dialysis I can live my life?" They were looking miserable, financially drained off and suffering beyond comparison. No one to turn to, it was a pathetic feeling of experience. These patients were physically suffering, spiritually dull, financially drained off, nothing to look forward to, with only one hope that if anyone could give them a kidney, they want to live more years! Is it be possible? Any angels come their way and do this miracle. We take for granted when all our body functions work well. I felt solidarity and concern for these patients; I felt the limitedness and helplessness. I felt how precious life is if it is lived well. Health is wealth and is a supreme gift we enjoy without realizing it until one day we lose it. We feel value of it at a time when it is too late.

Therefore, I thought of writing on this topic that how important it is to have kidney transplanted and give the eternal joy to someone who is waiting in expectation.

I feel that all the nurses who are working in the dialysis unit to be a sign of hope, joy and bring some solace to this pathetic condition. These nurses too need added strength to be with the patients round the clock, getting at times no reward and satisfaction of work being done, as there may not be successful recovery, as long-term dialysis patients keep coming and day by day getting weak and feeble and for most patients it becomes their last journey. They come repeatedly for dialysis and at the end, death awaits them. How much can a family support them? The loneliness and social stigma attached to it, and pain beyond the physical and mental suffering.

The book has two sections — Section 1 is covered in 15 chapters and Section 2 in 15 chapters. Both the sections have a number of figures which makes each topic interesting and valuably unique and distinct.

Section 1 gives the information and knowledge about **artificial kidney dialysis (AKD)** unit. It covers the topics—definition and principles of HD, process of admission, different job responsibility, procedure and nurse's responsibility, job description of technician, dialysis fluids and water treatment system, vascular care, guideline instructions and management of risk factors, blood transfusion, complications of HD, hospital printed records and equipment in the unit, routine activities, diet advice for HD, organ donation and kidney transplant, and a glance on the urinary system.

Section 2 deals with **operation theater (OT)** techniques and surgical aspects. This also is an important area could be explored by a nurse for a specialization. It contains topics like three phases of surgery, skin preparation for surgery, preparing an operation theater trolley, sterile technique, positioning client for surgery, endoscopy, anesthesia, thoracentesis, performing neonatal resuscitation and chest compression, preoperative check list, medical instruments, infection control, understanding nursing profession and new research in surgery, and burns wound management (medically and surgically).

The nurse has to follow all the principles and nursing intervention for maintaining a sterile field. She also has a role in cleaning, disinfection and sterilization of items, instruments, and quality management, competency, and developing standards of nursing care.

The change is associated with tremendous speed. If we have to survive and keep pace with it, we have to bring competitive change in our thinking, feelings, behavior and system of functioning. We have to adopt new technology, new knowledge and skills.

Keeping these sentiments and feelings at heart the importance of the subject, I have prepared this book with two sections. I believe that nursing fraternity will welcome it.

Cecilia Correia

Acknowledgments

I am humbled before Almighty God of wisdom and knowledge who has inspired me in my writing work. I am grateful to all those people who have made me what I am today with their contribution, directly or indirectly.

I am also privileged and honored by CBS Publishers & Distributors Pvt Ltd. I am happy to know that Mr. Satish Kumar Jain (CMD), who is a great visionary and dynamic person, established CBS PD in 1972. May he live in the hearts of all knowledge- and wisdom-thirsty souls. I deeply believe that what we do for ourselves dies with us, what we do for others remains immortal. I salute to him with his committed and dedicated team. I am grateful to Mr Ramesh Krishanamachari who introduced to me CBSPD, the leading publishing-cum-book distribution organization, which has grown as an international organization known for quality textbooks in medical sciences and technology.

May this book bring peace and good health to those who read it.

Cecilia Correia

Contents

Abbreviations

AKD	Artificial kidney dialysis
AKI	Acute kidney injury
ARF	Acute renal failure
AV Fistula	Arteriovenous fistula
CAVH	Continuous arteriovenous hemofiltration
CFU	Colony forming unit
CRF	Chronic renal failure
CRRT	Continuous renal replacement therapy
CVC	Central venous catheter
ESRD	End stage of renal disease
EU	Endotoxin unit
FBV	Fiber bundle valve
FFP	Fresh frozen plasma
HD	Hemodialysis
HF	Hemoperfusion
IUF	Isolated ultrafiltration
MRD	Medical record department
OT	Operation theatre
PPE	Personal protective equipment
RO	Reverse osmosis
SCUF	Slow continuous ultrafiltration
UF	Ultrafiltration

Introduction

Modern Dialysis Machines Unit needs to be carefully planned and headed by experienced Nephrologists and adequately staffed with trained, committed, caring technicians and nurses. Nephrologists should be available round the clock to supervise all patients as the Unit runs three to four shifts every day. Most of the chronic renal failure patients undergo dialysis three times a week (Mon/Wed/Fri or Tue/Thu/Sat) to ensure optimal benefits. Dialysis for acute renal failure patients is done as and when needed.

Procedures done in AKD are hemodialysis, plasma pheresis, subclavian jugular line, femoral line insertion, blood collection for laboratory investigations, blood transfusion, AV fistula dressing, and others (covered in Section 1).

Dialysis is a dynamic process. Little overlook can cause serious consequences. Condition of the patient before, during and just after the session of dialysis is important to recognize because it has direct bearing on patient's immediate as well as long-term prognosis.

As soon as the patient comes in, his vitals (blood pressure, temperature, pulse rate, respiratory rate and weight) are recorded. The concerned staff informs duty doctor/senior staff, if any parameters are below or above the range. Dialysis is not started unless the nephrologist sees that patient.

Patient's intradialytic weight gain, access condition and complains are also recorded before starting. Dialysis session's length, rate of heparinization, amount of ultrafiltration, blood flow rate, ultrafiltration rate/profile and dialysate composition are set and mentioned clearly according to the nephrologist's prescription and patient's conditions. Number of dialyzer and tubing reuse also mentioned.

During dialysis hourly and as and when required the blood pressure is recorded, all intradialytic events are mentioned.

After completion of dialysis all vitals are recorded once more. All medications given during or immediately after the dialysis are written clearly. Before the patient goes back, senior staff/nephrologist sign the form after checking all details.

Keeping records of patient's complete medical history is very important. The information is recorded in different forms by the attending doctor. It not only provides vital information in cases of emergencies but also helps in prognostication, rehabilitation and research-related activities. Medical history, recorded in three different forms, is obtained by attending duty doctor or senior technician or senior nursing staff. Once treating nephrologist sees and verifies, it is kept in patient's folder.

Form 1 : Medical history
Form 2 : Treatment/drug history
Form 3 : Investigation chart

It is mandatory for staff to obtain a signed consent about dialysis and related procedure from patient or in case of minor/mentally retarded/handicapped patients, from their immediate caregiver. Without complete consent of patient or immediate caregiver (in special cases), no procedure including dialysis, IV cannulation, ascites tapping, injection or vaccine administration in dialysis unit is allowed.

Section 2 deals with operation theater (OT) techniques. This section contains 15 chapters in nutshell which will give the overall knowledge to the nurse interested in learning the OT techniques and surgical aspects.

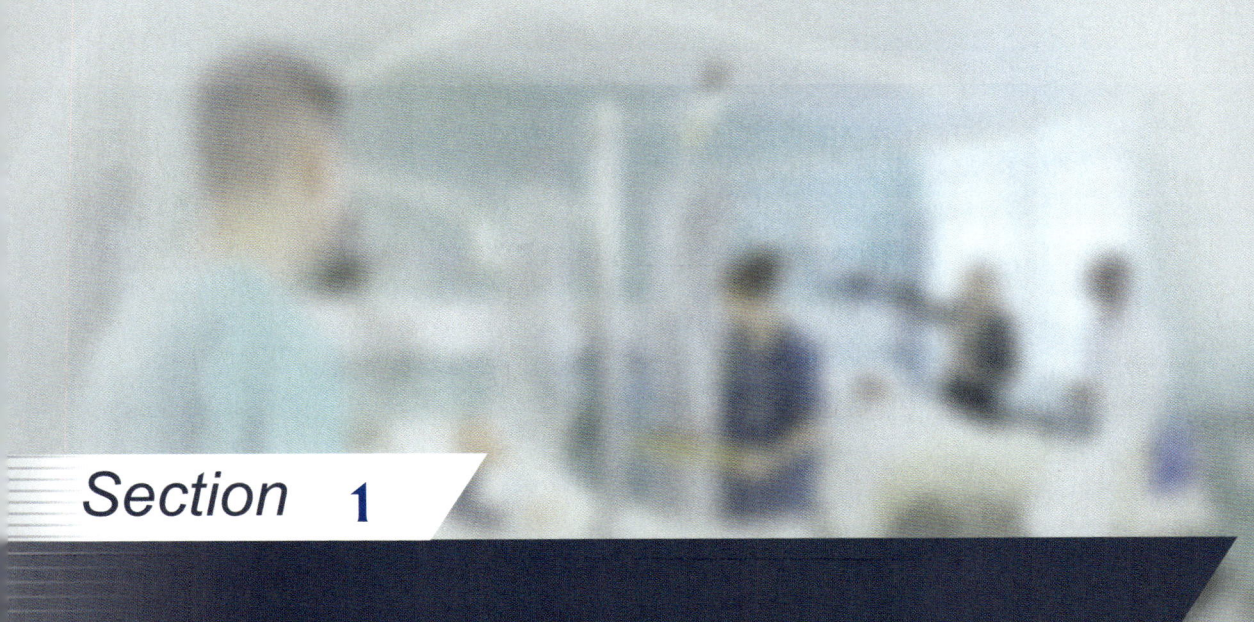

Artificial Kidney Dialysis Unit

Chapter 1

Definition, Purpose and Principles of Hemodialysis

Dialysis is a physicochemical process, which refers to the separation of two solutions by a semipermeable membrane through which water, and some solutes may pass. Dialysis is a therapeutic procedure used in acute and chronic renal failure to lower the blood level of metabolic waste products and toxic substances and to correct abnormal electrolyte and fluid imbalance.

A regular dialysis regimen has prolonged the life of many patients with chronic renal failure. It has permitted many of them to continue in their jobs and be independent, useful members of the society.

Hospital dialysis units have increased in numbers in resent years, yet the number of patients that can be treated is still limited.

Hemodialysis is the more efficient method of dialysis but it is more complex procedure, which requires more equipment that are sophisticated.

Hemodialysis (HD) is a treatment required for patients with end stage of renal disease (ESRD) or acute renal failure (ARF), which is loss of renal function.

DEFINITION OF HEMODIALYSIS

In hemodialysis, the client's blood flows through vascular catheters, passes by the dialysis solution in an external machine. It invokes diverting toxin laden blood from the client into a dialyzer and then returning the clean blood to the client.

Hemodialysis is a process of filtering the patient's blood by passing it through a dialyser (commonly known as artificial kidney), that filters accumulated waste products, excess body water, electrolytes and acid from the blood. The clean filtered blood is returned back into the patient's body.

PRINCIPLES OF HEMODIALYSIS

Physical properties of behavior of solvents and Solutions are used to purify the blood from unwanted substances. The blood, which has higher concentration of unwanted substances, is allowed to come in the contact of a solution, which does not have any of those substances at all. The concentration differences between two solutions (blood and dialysate) leads to the diffusion, osmosis and ultra-filtration and ultimately reduces the burden of unwanted substances in the blood.

PURPOSE OF HEMODIALYSIS

1. To provide adequate dialysis to clients
2. To ensure that all dialysis staff follow the standard policy
3. To prolong the life span of kidney failure patients and prevent mortality
4. To extract toxic nitrogenous waste substances from the blood

Figures 1.1 to 1.4 will explain the complex procedure diffusion, osmosis and ultrafiltration of the hemodialysis

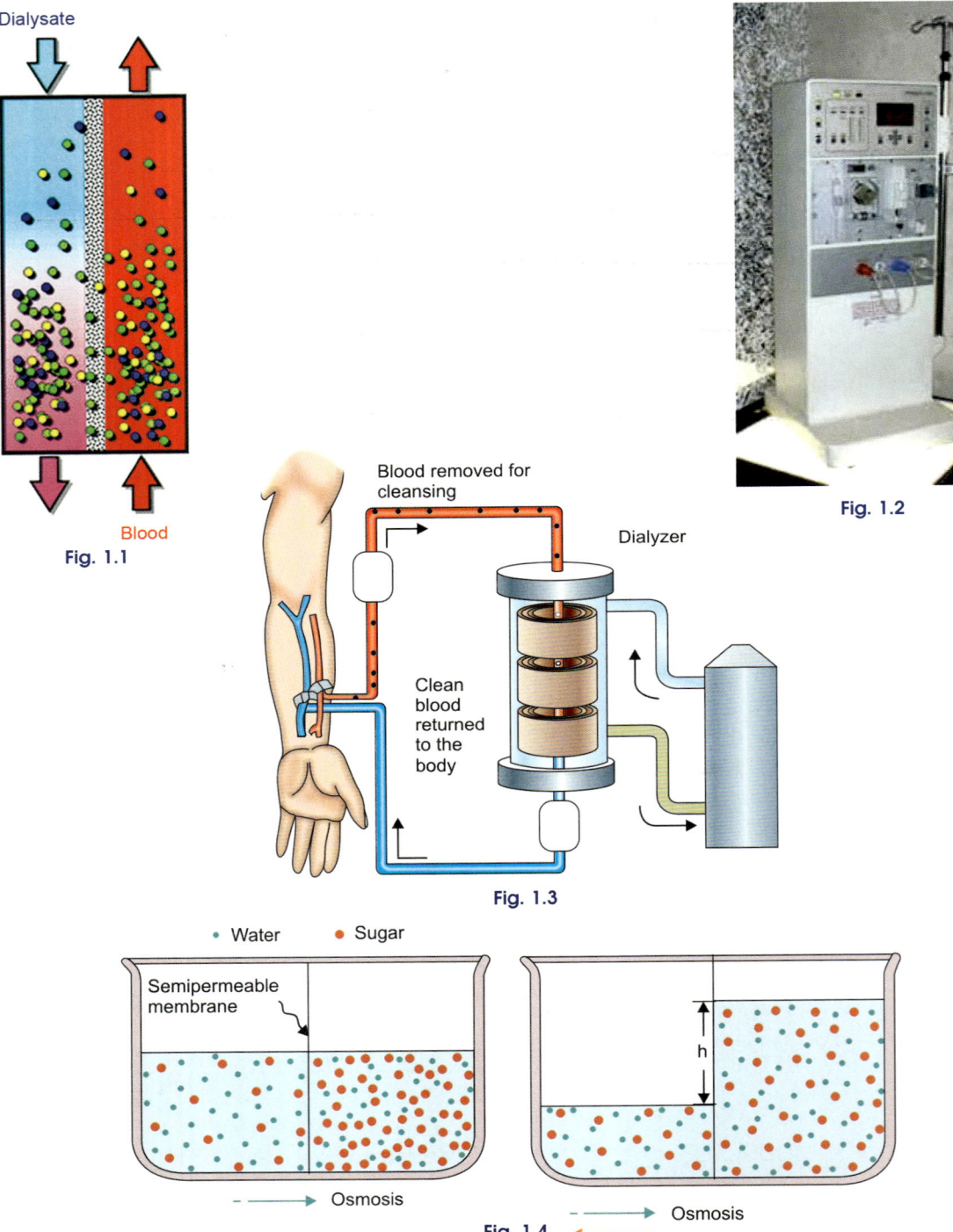

Dialysate

Blood

Fig. 1.1

Fig. 1.2

Blood removed for cleansing

Dialyzer

Clean blood returned to the body

Fig. 1.3

● Water   ● Sugar

Semipermeable membrane

h

Osmosis

Osmosis

Fig. 1.4

Figs 1.1 to 1.4: Diffusion, osmosis and ultrafiltration

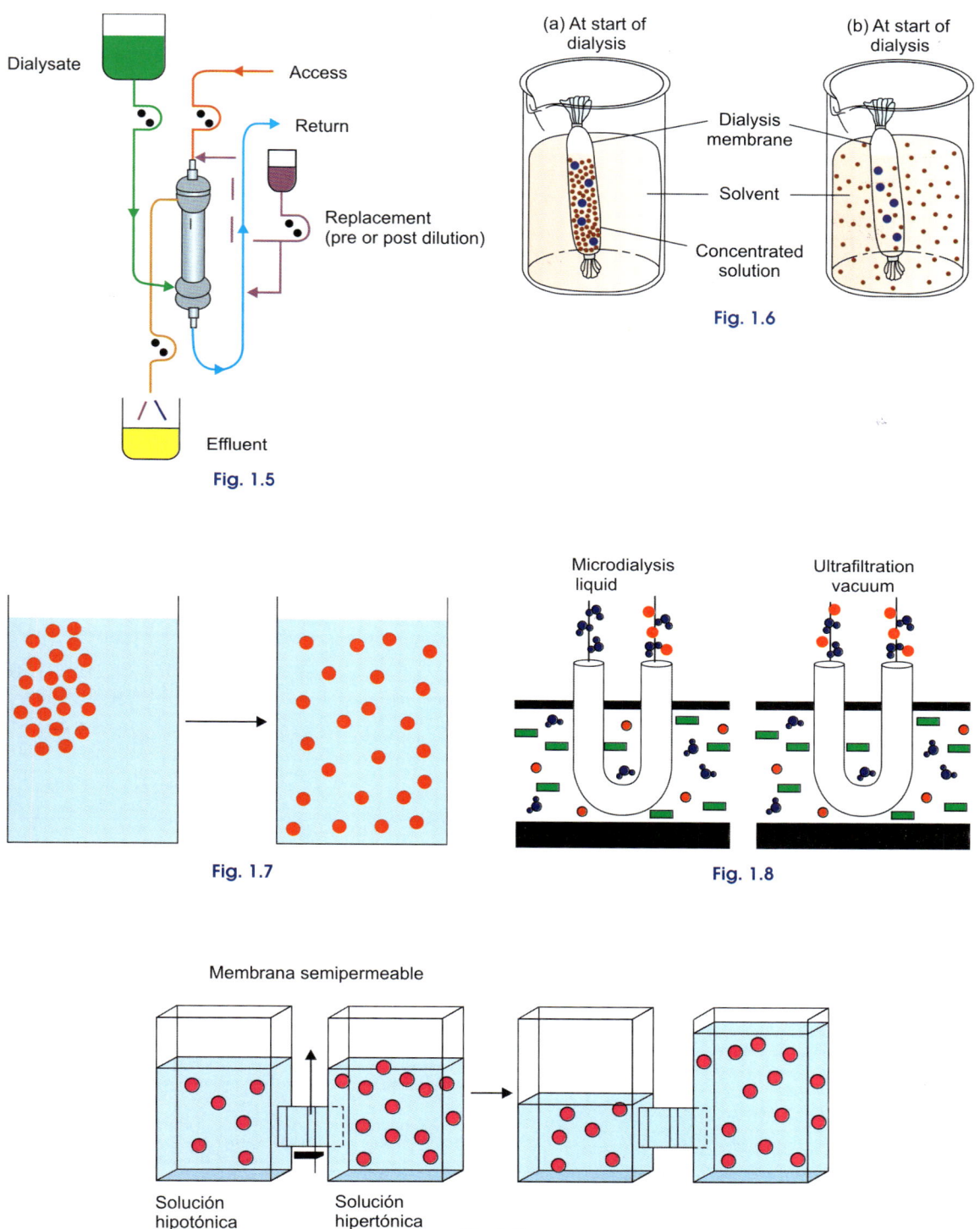

Dialysate

Access

Return

Replacement
(pre or post dilution)

Effluent

Fig. 1.5

(a) At start of
dialysis

(b) At start of
dialysis

Dialysis
membrane

Solvent

Concentrated
solution

Fig. 1.6

Fig. 1.7

Microdialysis
liquid

Ultrafiltration
vacuum

Fig. 1.8

Membrana semipermeable

Solución
hipotónica

Solución
hipertónica

Fig. 1.9

Figs 1.5 to 1.9: Procedure of osmosis, diffusion and ultrafiltration thus satisfactory biochemical control

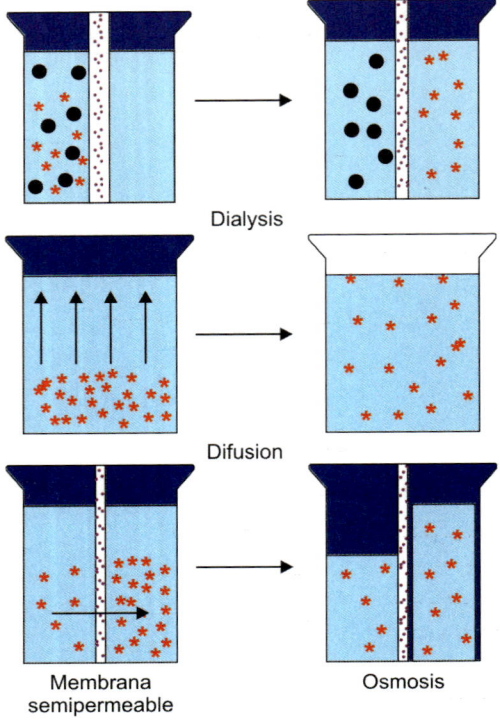

Fig. 1.10: Dialysis, diffusion and osmosis

5. To maintain fluid and electrolyte balance in the body.
6. To maintain acid–base balance (less commonly to remove ingested toxins and for drug overdose)
7. To standardize the process of dialysis for each patient coming in the dialysis unit.

Purpose of services is to take care of all the patients who need dialysis services for various medical reasons.

SCOPE of HD

1. Providing continuous dialysis care to all CKD stage 5 (ESRD) patients.
2. Providing urgent dialysis support to AKI (acute kidney injury) patients.
3. Providing dialysis for non renal indications like-fluid overload, acidosis, electrolytes; imbalance, drug overdose and poisoning.

4. Providing various modes of dialysis according to patient's condition, e.g. SLED (slow low efficiency dialysis) SCUF (slow continuous ultrafiltration) IUF (isolated ultra filtration) HF (hemoperfusion) HDF (hemodifiltration), etc. which can improve overall quality of life of all chronic renal failure patients.
5. In addition, provide health education to the patients and their relatives.
6. To educate dialysis staff through regular interaction and classes.

Indication of HD

1. CKD stage 5
2. AKI grade 3

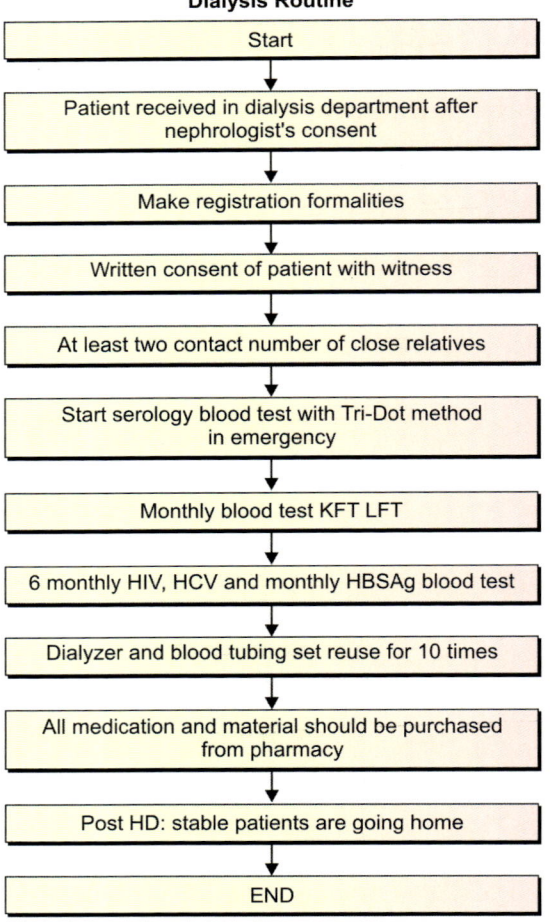

3. Acute or chronic renal failure
4. Hyperkalemia
5. Hypercalcemia
6. Intractable acidosis
7. Pulmonary edema
8. Fluid overload
9. Uremic pericarditis
10. Neuropathy
11. Encephalopathy
12. Gastritis
13. Bleeding
14. Drug overdose and poisoning.

Nurses responsible for the care of patients receiving dialysis require specialized preparation. Dialysis is a complex therapeutic procedure used to correct a life threatening body dysfunction, which needs the concerns of the renal patient and family. It is natural that the patient and family will be concerned and react. It is likely to have many implications, knowing that the disease has progressed to this stage and that life becomes dependent upon the procedure is extremely threatening. Severe anxiety may be manifested due to concern for the future and life expectancy. Acceptance may be difficult to some patients and they may manifest resentment followed by depression. Treatment may curtail his role in business, it may mean changing his occupation or giving up employment or working part time which may cause both social and economic changes for family members. Special diet requirements and transport to and from the dialysis unit may incur worrisome additional expense. It is important for the nurse to be willing listener and encourage patient and family. An understanding of their situation and recognition of their reactions are essential to providing the appropriate support and planning care, and in assisting them to accept the necessary modifications. A positive attitude on the part of the health care team promotes realistic patient and family acceptance and adaptation.

Chapter 2

Process of Admission and AV Fistula

PURPOSE

To facilitate smooth functioning of unit and effective coordination among patients, physicians, administrating, nursing and the AKD staff.

SCOPE

Minimizing patient's discomfort and avoiding unnecessary wait.

PROCEDURE

Nephrologists see the patient, provide written instructions to the patient, briefs him/her about the procedure and addresses his/her queries, concerns and doubts related to dialysis.

All outpatients having written instructions from nephrologists.

Nephrologists see all patients who come to ER/casualty. After nephrologist prescription casualty staff inform dialysis unit.

When a patient comes to the unit, a senior Nursing staff receives that patient. Receiving staff checks for all below mentioned things:

1. Nephrologists written prescription
2. Dialysis bill
3. Make a dialysis file.
4. Note down BP, pulse, temperature and general condition.
5. Fill the dialysis file with all mandatory details. This includes past and present medical history, drugs history, vaccination details, and status of the access
6. Check serology (HIV, HEP B/HEP C), CBC, RFT and blood group
7. Take written consent for dialysis and other procedures
8. Handover the patient to the senior dialysis technician.

The senior dialysis technician then

1. Explains patient about dialysis and related procedures
2. Addresses patient's fear, anxiety and concerns
3. Rechecks dialysis file, completed by nursing staff
4. Informs concern nephrologists about patient's condition, also inform administrative head, RMO

In charge and the dietician

5. Initiates dialysis
6. Assigns a nursing staff and a attended to take care of patient during dialysis.
7. Instruct a junior technician to monitor carefully and Note down all intradialytic events.
8. In case of any dialysis related complications, informs RMO on duty immediately.
9. Guides Junior technicians during termination of dialysis
10. Makes sure that all post-dialysis injections are given by assigned nursing staff.

11. Put his signature on the case paper after carefully rechecking all entry
12. Informs patient and his relatives about next dialysis timing, precaution before coming for dialysis and handover the dialysis education material.

Senior nursing staff that includes plans regular scheduler for investigations

1. *Monthly:* CBC, RFT, electrolytes with CA and PO_4
2. *Every 3rd month:* Serology, iron profile, glycosylated HB (for diabetic patient), lipid profile
3. *Yearly:* Intact PTH, antihepatitis B AB titer, ECG, 2D ECHO, chest X-ray.

PROCEDURE

Diffusion

Solute movement between blood and dialysate compartments through the dialyser membrane occurs by diffusion. Diffusion is a process of movement of solutes from higher concentration in the blood to an area of lower concentration is the dialysate across the semi-permeable membrane.

Ultrafiltration

Water moving under high pressure to an area of lower pressure. Water is pushed out of the dialyser membrane by pressure gradient between blood and dialysate compartments of dialyser. This drags along with it some solutes in the blood. Ultrafiltration also helps to remove excess body water.

Hemodialysis process has three essential aspects

Obtaining patient's blood with a good speed and directing it towards the dialyser.

Preparing machine and dialyser to receive the blood and remove unwanted substances in a desired way. Sending back the purified blood.

Termination of dialysis, washing of dialyzer and cleaning/preparation of machines for next session of dialysis.

Good blood flow which is an essential prerequisite for dialysis can be obtained either by permanent or temporary access. Permanent accesses are AV fistula and graft and temporary access is a 'double luman' dialysis catheter. Temporary access can be put in internal jugular, sub-clavian or femoral vein.

Central Venous Catheter

Immediate access to the patient's circulation for acute hemodialysis is achieved by inserting a double-lumen catheter in to the internal jugular, subclavian or femoral vein. Internal jugular vein is the most preferred one. Catheter can be used for 4–6 weeks in jugular vein, 2–4 weeks in subclavian vein and 1–2 weeks in femoral vein.

Arteriovenous (AV) Fistula

A fistula is created surgically to improve the blood flow in the easily accessible veins of the upper arm, by joining an artery to an adjacent vein. Preferred sites for fistula creation are either radio-cephalic near the wrist or basilo-cephalic in the forearm.

Fistula takes 1–6 months to mature. The patient is encouraged to perform exercises to increase the size of these vessels (i.e. squeezing a rubber ball).

Minimum recommend waiting is 4 weeks prior to cannulation of the fistula.

Hemodialysis with an AV fistula involves the insertion of two needles into the vein. One needle is inserted at least 2 cm above the fistula and is connected to the outflow or arterial line of the dialyser. The second needle is inserted 3–4 cm above the outflow needle and is connected to the tube that returns the blood from the dialyser. Blood flows out from the distal needle through the dialyser and back into the patient via the proximal needle. A single needle technique using a Y-connector to permit alternate arterial and venous flow may be used. The limb in which an AV fistula is developed should not normally be used in talking blood pressure or blood specimens, as either may jeopardize their patency.

An arteriovenous (AV) shunt is established by exposing an artery and an adjacent vein an implanting a cannula in each. The ends of the cannula tubes are brought through the skin and are joined by a short connecting tube. The cannula and tubing are of inert synthetic materials so that reactions are avoided. The incisions are sutured around the tubes and a sterile dressing and bandage are applied. To start dialysis the shunt-tubing is clamed and then the connecting tube on the AV shunt is removed; the arterial cannula is connected to the inflow line of the dialyser and the venous cannula is attached to the outflow dialyser tube to the tube which returns the blood to the patient.

Arteriovenous Graft

It can be created by subcutaneously interposing a biologic, semibiologic or synthetic graft placed between a artery and vein. Most commonly used synthetic graft material is expanded polytetrafluoroethylene. This created in case of patient vessels are not suitable for fistula (common sites are forearm, upper arm, upper thigh). Grafts can be Cannulated in 2–3 weeks after placement once the subcut tunnel heals.

Steps

Patient arrival: Every patient coming to dialysis unit is received as per the schedule and made comfortable. Relative is guided to visitor's lobby.

Check the payment voucher before taking the patient for dialysis.

Patient assessment: Baseline-vital signs, weight, neurological status, physical assessment, fluid and electrolyte status.

Observe graft, fistula, catheter insertion site for signs and symptoms of infection.

Check the catheter for patency.

Before initiating hemodialysis, enquire about patient's wellbeing in the interdialytic period and any relevant medical history such as fever, diarrhea, bleeding from any site and cough should be noted and informed to the nephrologists.

ACCESS CANNULATION

- Take consent.
- Keep patient in a comfortable position that will facilitate optimal blood flow through the catheter/fistula.
- Wash hands thoroughly.
- Place a sterile towel.
- Prepare the site by wiping with betadine in a circular manner.
- Prime the dialyser tubing and put it into circulation.
- Wear sterile gloves and mask. Select the site.
- Grasp butterfly wings or hub of fistula needle between thumb and index finger of dominant hand.
- Remove needle guard.
- Hold the skin.
- With dominant hand, insert needle at a 45° angle to the skin. Arterial needle is inserted first. It is placed 3 cm away from AV anastomosis and directed towards the anastomosis. Venous needle is placed more proximal, at least 5 cm away from the arterial needle directed towards the heart.
- Remove tourniquet before inserting normal saline or heparin.
- Aspirate blood, infuse flush solution and re-clamp catheter.
- Secure needle with adhesive tape over insertion site.
- Discard soiled material in appropriate receptacle.
- Wash hands.
- Place yellow band on the AV fistula hand or the hand, which is preserved for AV fistula.

ACCESSING A CATHETER

1. Wash hands thoroughly.
2. Prepare a sterile field, sterile container, dressing materials

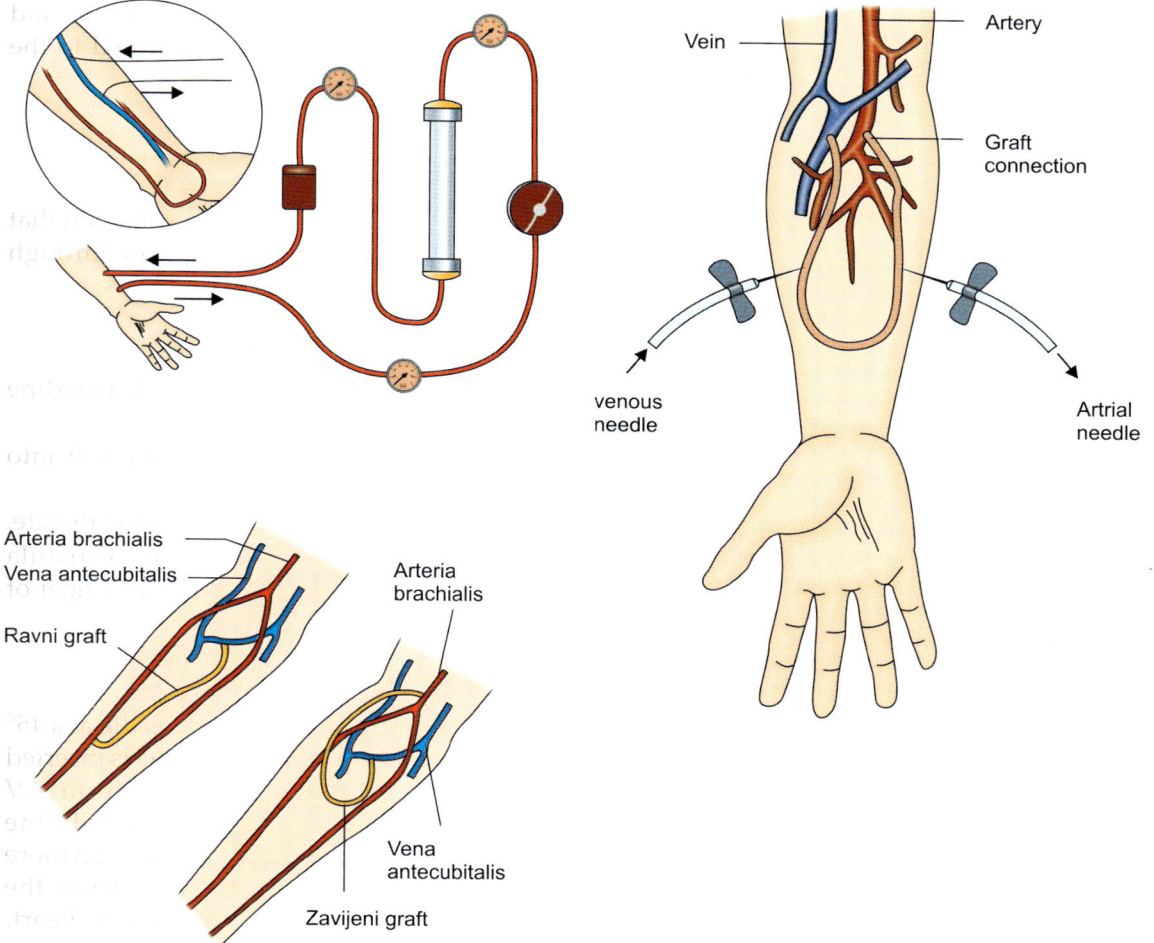

Vein

Artery

Graft connection

venous needle

Artrial needle

Arteria brachialis
Vena antecubitalis

Ravni graft

Arteria brachialis

Vena antecubitalis

Zavijeni graft

Fig. 2.1: An internal arteriovenous fistula is created by a side to side anastomosis of the artery and vein

3. Prepare flush solution.
4. Remove dressing.
5. Discard soiled dressing.
6. Wash hands.
7. Wear sterile gown, gloves, mask and goggles.
8. Clean the arterial and venous ends of the catheter with alcohol/chlorhexidine.
9. Remove cap from arterial hub of catheter and aspirate 3 cc of blood close the slide clamp, remove syringe and discard.
10. Same way aspirate venous blood
11. Soak pads in betadine and clean connector site.
12. Remove flush syringe and attach arterial line to the dialyses machine securely to the arterial limb.
13. Check if all connections are complete.
14. Tape connections securely.

INITIATION OF HEMODIALYSIS

1. Attach 'A' line to the 'A' needle and release the clamp
2. Drain out the saline. When the blood reaches the 'V' chamber stops the pump, clamp the 'V' line and attach to the 'V' needle.
3. Release the clamp and start the pump

4. Remove gloves and discard in the white liner.
5. Adjust blood flow rate to 150–200 ml/minute.
6. Adjust the blood level in the arterial and venous drip chamber.
7. Patient receives heparin infusion as per parameters.
8. Slowly increase the pump speed
9. Set arterial/venous alarm parameters.
10. Set the UF time
11. Document the vital parameters (hourly), start time, pump speed, UF rate and heparinization (10,000 IU per session of dialysis for each patient, specific cases will be decided by nephrologist)
12. Monitor the patient ½/1 hourly depending on the condition of the patient and document in the dialysis flow sheet.
13. Injection erythropoitin, iron or vitamin to be given as per the nephrologists order.

TERMINATION

1. Wash hands, wear gloves
2. Turn off the heparin infusion before ½ hr of termination.
3. Decrease the blood flow 150 ml/min
4. Confirm re-infusion mode
5. Clamp the arterial tubing attached to patient and the blood pump.

6. Disconnect the tubing from vascular access and obtain blood samples for lab studies if advised.
7. Clear the blood from the tubing's and dialyser with saline until rinse back is clear.
8. Turn of the blood pump
9. Clamp venous access if using a CVC (central venous catheter) and flush with heparin.
10. When fistula needle is used, remove both needles from access site, one at a time using a sterile pad apply moderate pressure.
11. Dispose soiled material as per IC policy.
12. Document the vital parameters, finish time, UF rate and heparinization, weight, post-dialysis collection if any and medications administered.

DISINFECTION OF THE DIALYSIS MACHINE

In between patient, water rinse is done for 10 minute.

At the end of the last shift every day, 5% sodium hypochlorite rinse is given for 10 min and is preserved for 4 hours, and then water rinse is given for 30 months.

On every saturday 4% formalin rinse is given for 15–20 months and then preserved for 24 hrs followed by water rinse.

Clean the exterior of the machine with Bacilloid spary.

Chapter 3

Job Responsibility and Staffing Pattern

Staffing pattern of AKD department.

Unit can be comprised of following members.

Chief Nephrologists

Technicians and staff nurses dialysis unit (senior technician, junior technician)

Attendant (ward boys–ward girls)

Nephrologist's job responsibility towards patient oriented is as follows:

Each hospital has there own policy description to be followed:

1. Patient assessment (examination, investigation)
2. Formulation of treatment plan
3. Provide written instructions to the staff about treatment plan
4. Patient and relative counselling (procedure, diet and medicines)
5. Putting temporary access, creating fistula
6. Ensure availability during procedure
7. Inventory-check all records at least twice/month
8. Medication related—prescription of medication, providing written instruction to the nursing staff about dose duration/site/precaution, educate patient and staff about all possible effects and side effects related to drugs being given, check all records at least once/week.
9. Smooth functioning of the unit
10. Explaining department policy and procedures to the new staff
11. Making duty roaster for technicians and arranging staff for emergency and on call duty.
12. Periodic checking of all registers maintained in the unit.
13. Supervision of technicians/nursing staff
14. Preparation of reports on department performance and reporting/updating the director.

Patient oriented job responsibilities of nurse:
1. Patient assessment
2. Patient and relative counselling (procedure, diet and medicines)
3. Initiation of dialysis and termination
4. Updating the medication chart according to consultant and nephrologists orders
5. Handling complications during the process (if any) and informing the consultant and nephrologists
6. Looking after patient schedule of viral markers and vaccinations
7. Inventory—regular checking of stock
8. Medication—regular checking of medicines stock (dressing trolley and crash card). Department—cleanliness in the department
9. Maintenance of dialysis machines
10. Skill sets required by a nurse for Technical know how are:
    a. Basic operation of the dialysis machine

   b. Rinsing the machine with chemicals and water

   c. Intermittent management of dialysis

   d. Reprocessing the dialyzer and tubing for next use

11. Basic knowledge of hospital information systems

12. To be alert of comfort level of patients, emergency care and management

13. Develop interpersonal skills—excellent communication skills with patients and relatives patient and courteous

14. Health education

15. Psychological support to patient and relatives

16. *Basic emergency training:* Requires training in BLS, ACLS and emergencies specific to dialysis

Other general job responsibilities of AKD nurse:

 a. Maintaining flowchart

 b. Maintain investigation chart

 c. Maintain dialysis payment book

 d. Maintain registration book

 e. Daily inventory book

 f. CSSD book

 g. Three monthly expiry medication record book

 h. Communication book

 i. Consumable record book

 j. Replacement book

 k. Investigation book

 l. Fumigation record book

 m. To keep all clients record for medical record department (MRD)

 n. Regular indent of pharmacy and stores

 o. Maintaining OPD, IPD registers and dialysis tubing consumption book

General Guidelines

1. All breaks in dialysis precautions require an incident report, and evaluation to determine future preventive strategies and possible disciplinary action, which might occur through negligence

2. Keep a dialysis register in which details of clients can be entered

3. Anticipate the kind of client contact and use the appropriate personal protective equipment (PPE)

4. Know the limitations of the personal protective equipment you are using, when the equipment can protect you, and when it cannot HBsAg + VE, HCV+VE clients to be taken in isolation machine dedicated to client

Do not perform any invasive procedure or assess BP on AV fistula hand.

Responsibilities of ward attendant towards patient:

5. Patient assistance

6. Patient movement (wheelchair)

7. Providing patients with eatables (tea/ coffee, snacks)

8. Aiding patient in bowel movements

9. Inventory: Pick up of materials from stores and pharmacy

10. Cleanliness in the department

11. Cleaning of biomedical equipment

12. Bed making

13. Delivering soiled linen to laundry

14. Bringing and delivery materials to CSSD

15. Skill sets required—safety management of patient

16. Alert to comfort level of patients

17. *Interpersonal skills:* Good communication skills with patients and relatives

Chapter 4

Procedure and Nurse's Responsibility

Pre-dialysis Procedure: Nursing Responsibility

1. Keep the files, dialyzer, tubing in order of client as per schedule
2. Receive the client
3. Instruct/remind client to use the washroom
4. Take written consent from the client for Hemodialysis procedure
5. *Check the file of the client:* Last, date of dialysis, blood test BUN, creatinine levels (monthly checking), (Hb, RBS, every 6 months) weight, BP, and medications. Inform when his due date is. Record and maintain intake out-put chart
6. *In case of weight gain:* Double check, inform client (read out aloud), inform technician and RMO
7. Allot the bed to client, make the client to lie in comfortable position
8. Shave and clean the area before inserting needles
9. Do not use affected extremity for BP or venipuncture to prevent bruising, bleeding and risk for infection
10. Check the AV fistula site for bruit (auscultation) and thrill (palpating)
11. Assist the technician for catheter cleaning, dressing and needle cannulation:
    - Clean the fistula site with spirit and sterile green towel is kept under arm and cannulation is done
    - Artery and vein lines are connect and start HD
    - Give injection heparin bolus dose 2.500 IU and set 2.3 ml/hour set for 3 hours.

During Dialysis Procedure: Nursing Responsibility

1. Monitor TPR and B/P 1 hourly and as per need
2. Fistula is observed for bruit and thrill
3. Complete flowchart
4. Perform RBS when need
5. Observe for any adverse reaction (changes such as hypotension, hypoglycemia, hypothermia, shivering, chills, fever, vomiting, chest pain) during dialysis, if any change observed immediately consultant is notified. In case of need call RMO on duty
6. Staff nurse administer oral medication or injections as per nephrologist's order (avoid IM during dialysis procedure). SOS use venous line
7. After 2 hours provide tea and biscuits to the client
8. Administer injection interferon with 100 ml/N/S one hour before termination
9. Watch for any complication during dialysis and inform consultant

Post-dialysis Procedure:
Nursing Responsibility

1. Give post-dialysis injection (erythropoietin or antibiotic as ordered). Document the same in clients file.
2. Perform the dressing with aseptic technique, in case of jugular or femoral catheter.
3. Check and record in client's file and appointment card the details of BP, heart rate and post HD weight.
4. Attach the nurses notes record in clients file nursing (pre-during, post-GC)
5. Label the dialyzer unit
6. Check for S/S of infection at catheter exit site.
7. Practice universal precautions for all clients.
8. Post dialysis remove the fistula needles and give pressure on needle site with gauze pieces, apply antibiotic powder/ointment and tie with tourniquet.
9. Explain client to remove the tourniquet after 4–6 hours and in between watch for oozing.
10. See doctor immediately if the access site bleeds or catheter becomes dislodged.

Patient Education

1. Keep site and extremity warm, advise client to wash it daily.
2. Educated client and relatives' how to untie the tourniquet at home.
3. Doctor should be seen immediately if the access site bleeds or catheter becomes dislodged.
4. Avoid wearing constrictive clothing or ornaments, watch over the access site.
5. Avoid lifting/carrying heavy baggage.
6. Take regular medications as per advised by the doctor.
7. Perform routine investigations as per nephrologists order.

Attributes of Successful Nurse

1. Communication skills
2. Detail orientation
3. Competent
4. Commitment
5. Passion
6. Intuitive
7. Compassion
8. Flexibility/calm
9. Team spirit
10. Efficiency

Chapter 5

Technician's Job Description

1. Patient assessment
2. Patient and relative counselling (procedure, diet and medicines)
3. Initiation of dialysis and termination
4. Updating the medication chart according to consultant and nephrologists orders
5. Scheduling successive appointments for patients
6. Looking after due dates of bimonthly dialysis package and viral markers of patients.
7. Cannulation of AV fistula, graft catheter
8. Handling complications during the process (if any) and informing the consultant and nephrologist
9. Inventory—Indenting stock from main store and pharmacy
10. Regular checking of stock
11. Showing consumption of stock
12. Department—cleanliness in the department
13. Maintenance of dialysis machines
14. Checking the number of inpatient dialysis and coordinating for billing.
15. Explaining department policy and procedures to the new patients and arranging dialysis.
16. Making duty roaster for technicians and arranging staff for emergency and on call duty.
17. Arranging and coordination for linen and CSSD materials on a day to day basis.
18. Maintaining OPD, IPD registers and dialysis tubing consumption book.
19. Supervision of housekeeping/ward attendant
20. Preparation of reports on department performance and reporting/updating the general manager.
21. *Skill sets required:* Technical know-how—Basic operation of the dialysis machine
22. Rinsing the machine with chemicals and water
23. Intermittent management of dialysis
24. Reprocessing the dialyzer and tubing for next use
25. Temporary repair of emergency break down of machines (if within scope).
26. Basic knowledge of hospital information systems
27. Alertness-errors on the machine
28. Comfort level of patients
29. Interpersonal skills—excellent communication skills with patients and relatives patient and courteous.
30. Basic emergency training—requires training in BLS, ACLS and emergencies specific to dialysis.
31. Additional responsibilities—reporting to the general manager for patient problems, grievances, department problems.
32. In the absence of the executive officer, taking charge of the department.

GENERAL RESPONSIBILITY OF DIALYSIS TECHNICIAN TO MONITOR MACHINE

Prepare a schedule for next day.

Before the Procedure

Equipment (machine) preparation:
1. Prepare fresh bicarbonate dialysis solution
2. Give the machine reverse osmosis (RO) water rinse for 15 minutes
3. After rinse put the machine in the "test mode"
4. Drain the renaclean out of tubing and dialyzer
5. Prime the tubing and dialyzer with one liter normal saline
6. A + B part connected machine
7. T-1 test done

Patient Preparation

1. Identify the correct client
2. Explain procedure to the client
3. Wash hands
4. Wear gown
5. Wear clean gloves and wash with sterillium
6. Checking of fistula for bruit and thrill
7. Place towel on rubber sheet
8. Clean fistula with spirit
9. Cannulate the fistula hand and immobilize the needle by applying gauze with plaster.
10. Set the weight and time.
11. When machine is ready to connect the handset connection to dialyzer.
12. Connect the blood tubing to the client and start HD.

During the Procedure

1. Flush the blood compartment and dialysate compartment with Reverse Osmosis (RO) water
2. Rinse the blood compartment and dialysate compartment with RO water under PSI 15.20.

3. Observe and handle troubleshooters of dialysis machines.
4. Monitor venous pressure
5. Monitor arterial pressure
6. Monitor blood flow
7. Maintain and monitor transmembrane pressure
8. Check for clotting of tubing and dialyzer conductivity
9. Check air in the tubing and dialyzer
10. Check blood leak from the dialyzer and tubing
11. Inspect for clots, rupture, etc.
12. If any unusual change has been noticed in machine the same has to be communicated to the engineer/company

After the Procedure

1. Disinfect the tubing with Renaclean
2. Disinfect the dialyzer with Renaclean 4% and store for seven days for re-use till the client arrives in the next session.
3. Water analysis report and dialysis machine sample
4. Daily chlorine test to be done by the technician
5. After procedure—Rinse with RO water for 10 minuets
6. Priming—dialyzer and tubing to remove for chemical disinfectant (Renaclean)
7. Rinse the dialyzer and tubing with normal saline

Closing Hemodialysis (HD) by Technician

1. After the therapy time is over disconnect the arterial line from the client
2. Stop blood pump
3. Disconnect artery lines
4. Artery needle flushed with normal saline, and connect the saline with artery line tubing.
5. Start the blood pump and flush all blood from tubing and dialyzer with saline, and return blood to the client by "milking the tubing".

6. After returning the blood, disconnect the venous line from the client
7. Remove the clients AVF needle and apply pressure. Apply plaster or tourniquet and instruct the client to loose tunicate after 3–4 hours at home.

MONTHLY SERVICING, CLEANING AND TESTING

Responsibility of washing of dialyzer by technician

Servicing

1. Dialyzer container to be washed and kept ready monthly.
2. Dialysis machine servicing—four monthly—done by company people (four times a year)
3. Machine calibration—yearly—done by company
4. Pump servicing—three months—done by company, AMC company/annual maintenance service contract is followed (every two weeks regeneration softener is done, water analysis done every 6 months.)

Cleaning

1. Disconnect the handset connector
2. Remove the dialyzer and wash under pressure

3. Rinse with hot water and remove all blood clots.
4. Discard the hot water from the dialyzer and tubing, which are filled with disinfecting chemicals.
5. Dialyzer is washed and connected to reprocessing machine for disinfection
6. Monitor volume, and pressure.
   - This procedure is of 12 minutes. Then remove and keep in the box. After every HD machine is rinsed with water.
   - Weekly every saturday all machines with chemical Hypo-bleach cleaning done
   - Clean tank monthly (by maintenance department and supervisors)
   - Change filter
   - RO (reverse osmosis) water plant servicing done every 3 months
   - Membrane cleansing is performed every 2–3 month

Testing

1. Dialysis machine electrolyte test in lab done as per need
2. RO plant and dialysis machine water for culture test is done
   Endotoxins test done every 6 months
   Note: Each institution will have there own policy.

Chapter 6

Dialysis Fluid and Water Treatment System

Dialysis Catheter Care and Maintenance

Dialysis catheter lumens can be accessed to dialysis technicians only. Central venous access for dialysis is a safe, aseptic procedure. It must be used for infusion, medication and blood drawing only with a specific order from the nephrology team.

Contents in Dialysis Fluid

A-part contains: 1000 ml each

Potassium chloride	6.00 gms
Magnesium chloride	3.70 gms
Calcium chloride	8.10 gms
Sodium chloride	165.00 gms
Acetic acid	9.46 gms

Equivalents of ready to use Hemodialysis solution	2.20 mmol/l
K^+	0.50 mmol/l
Mg^{2+}	1.50 mmol/l
Ca^{2+}	136.00 mmol/l
Cl^-	103.00 mmol/l
CH_3COO^-	4.50 mmol/l
HCO_3	39.00 mmol/l

B-part contains

Sodium bicarbonate	66.00 gms
Sodium chloride	23.50 gms

Diluted in 10 liters of purified water

Reuse of Dialyser and Tubing Washing Method

Dialyser

1. Cleaning–flushing water into blood compartment and dialysis compartment of dialyser
   - Keep under 15 to 20 PSI water pressure for 10 to 15 minutes
   - Then rinse blood compartment by 2 to 3 liters of water, then dialysate compartment.
2. FBV (fiber bundle valve)
   If FBV is less then 80% then discard the dialyser
3. Filling dialyser with 4% Renaclean

Blood Tubing

- After termination of dialysis disconnect the tubing from the dialyser and then pass water through the tubing
- Thereafter pass 2% of hypochloride solution through the tubing
- 5 to 10 minutes hold time is allowed to enable all clots to be dissolved
- Connect arterial end of the blood tubing is then connected to the tap and allow 2 to 3 liters of water is allowed to flow
- The tube connects to the dialyser and filled with 4% Renaclean (10 liters: 400 ml Renaclean + 9600 RO water) = 4%

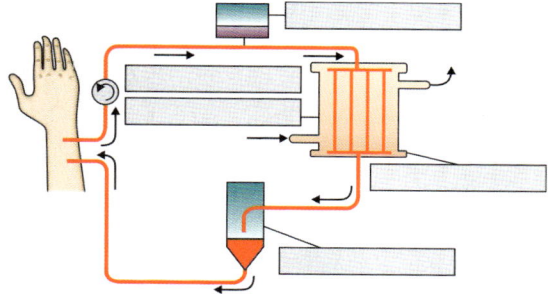

Fig. 6.1: Hemodialysis

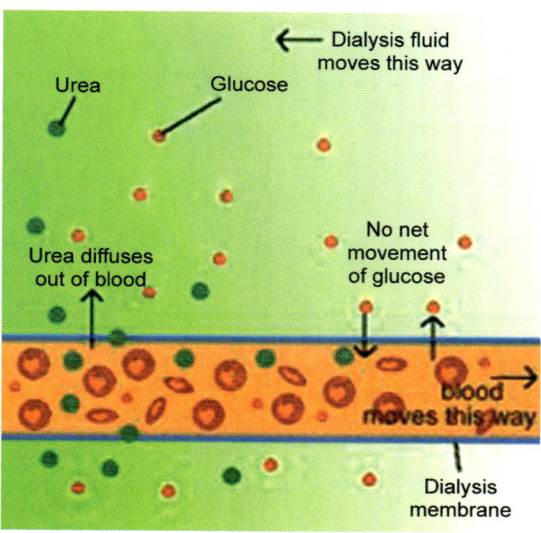

Fig. 6.3: Semipermeable membrane

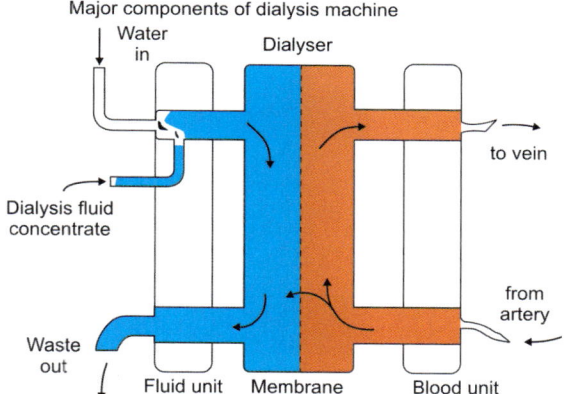

Fig. 6.2: Dialysis machine

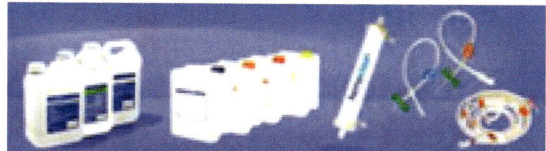

Fig. 6.4: Equipment for hemodialysis

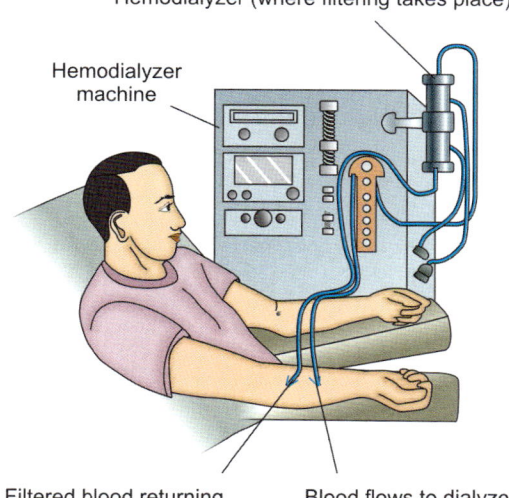

Fig. 6.5: Filtering during dialysis

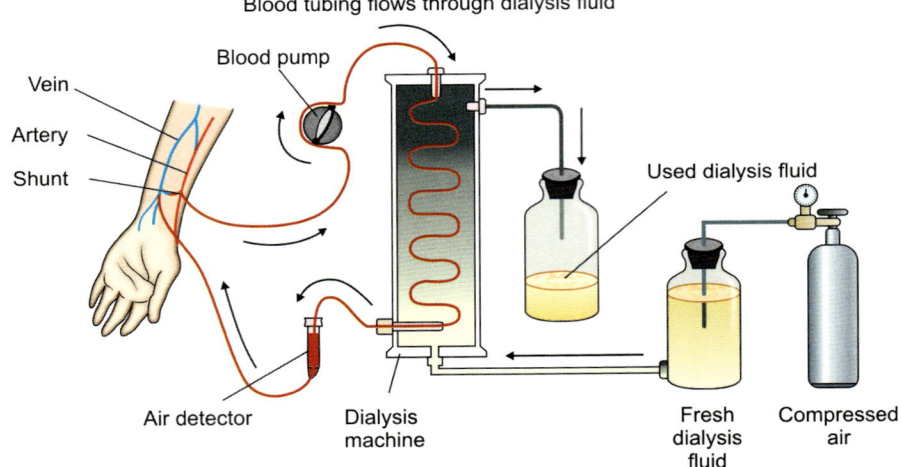

Fig. 6.6: Hemodialysis process

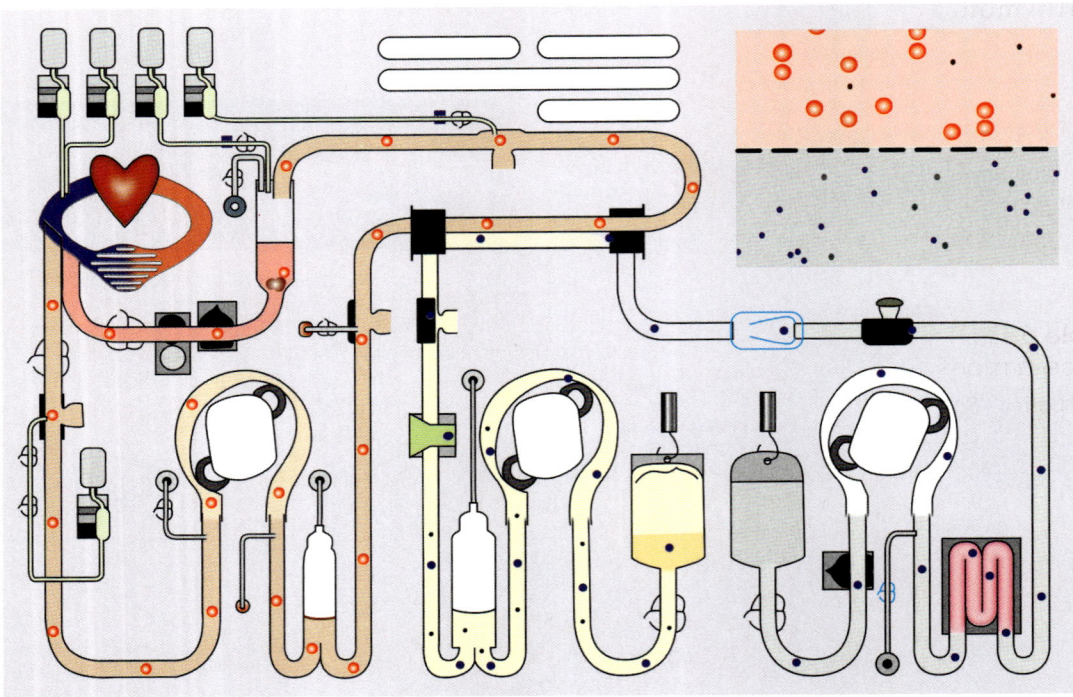

Fig. 6.7: Dialysis fluid and water treatment system

(Renaclean consists of hydrogen peroxide and per acetic acid) and its dwell time is 11 hours. It should be used within 7 days, and its dwell time is 24 hours.

Note: Tubing should be used only 10 to 15 times, and if it is damaged it should be discarded by filling it with 2% of hypochloride solution by cutting it at two different place.

Water Treatment System

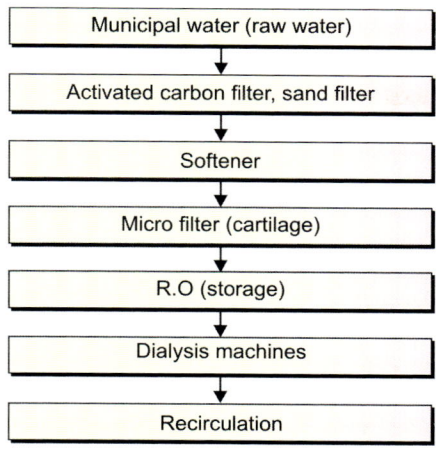

Activities of AKD

1. Machines servicing done regularly every 4th month (we have three different company machines such as Niprohemoclean solution used for it, Fresenius machine where citrosterl solution used, B-Brown machine citric acid solution is used)
2. Each morning machines are checked and then primed before putting client on dialysis
3. HCV machines are formalized time to time
4. All emergency drugs and trolleys are checked and updated daily. Central oxygen and suction are checked daily
5. Regular swabs and reverse osmosis (RO) and dialysate water are sent for colony forming units (CFU) and endotoxin unit (EU).

Note: Follow the hospital policy and manufactures instructions.

Table 6.1a: Dialysis machine and RO plant daily treatment policy

	Monday	Tuesday	Wednesday	Thursday	Friday	Saturday
Machine policy	Hemoclean or acetic acid (0.5%)	Hemoclean or formalize (con.37%)	Hemoclean or acetic acid	Hemoclean or formalize	Hemoclean or acetic acid	Bleach (sodium Hypo con. 5%)

Table 6.1b: Hot Disinfection done everyday for Fresenius machine and hemoclean done twice a month

RO policy	Softener rinse (plant water)	Softener regener (salt 7 kg water)	Softener rinse (plant water)	Softener regener (salt 7 kg water)	Softener rinse (plant water)	Softener regener (salt 7 kg water)

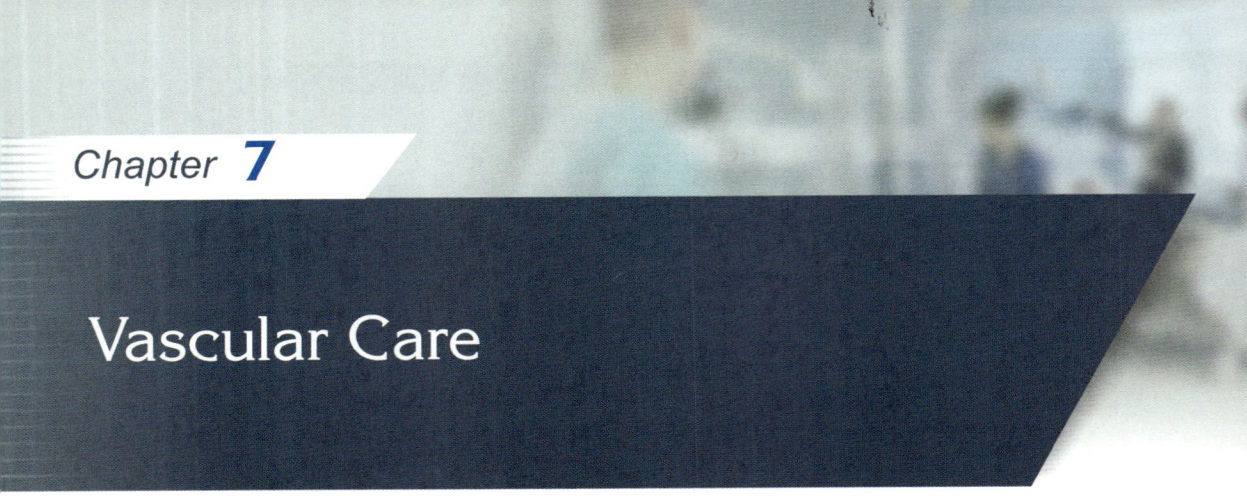

Chapter 7

Vascular Care

Purpose

To enhance the access patency rate and prevent access dysfunction. The use of aseptic technique and appropriate cannulation methods, the timing of fistula and graft cannulation, and early evaluation of immature fistulae are all factors that may prevent morbidity and may prolong the survival of permanent dialysis accesses.

Vascular care consists of:
1. Physical examination
2. Strict aseptic techniques
3. Cannulation
4. Prevention of dysfunction

Skin Preparation Techniques of Subcutaneous AV Accesses

Locate, palpate and inspect the needle cannulation site prior to skin preparation. Once the skin prep has been applied, wash with antibacterial soap or scrub and water. Cleanse the skin by 10% povidone iodine. Dialysis staff for cannulation should wear clean gloves. Gloves should be changed during any contamination at any time during cannulation procedure. Proper infection control measure followed for each patient.

CANNULATION

Fistulae are more likely to be useable when they meet the Rule of 6s characteristics: flow greater than 600 mL/min, diameter at least 0.6 cm, no more than 0.6 cm deep, and discernible margins.

If a fistula fails to mature by 6 wk, a fistulogram or other imaging study should be obtained to determine the cause of the problem.

Technique for Mature AVF

1. Cannulation—after skin preparation, apply a tourniquet to increase the venous pressure, and pull skin taut in opposite direction of needle insertion. Avoid excessive pressure to the Cannulation site to prevent flattering of the vessel. Stabilize but do not obliterate the vessel.

2. For easily palpated vessel, use approximately 25 inches angle with the bevel up. Arterial needle placement can be ante grade (up, in the direction of the blood flow) or retrograde (down, against the direction of the blood flow) the venous needle should always be in the same direction as the blood flow.

3. Once the vessel has been penetrated advance the needle slowly with cutting edge facing top of vessel and do not rotate axis.

4. Tape the needle at the same angle or one similar to the angle of insertion.

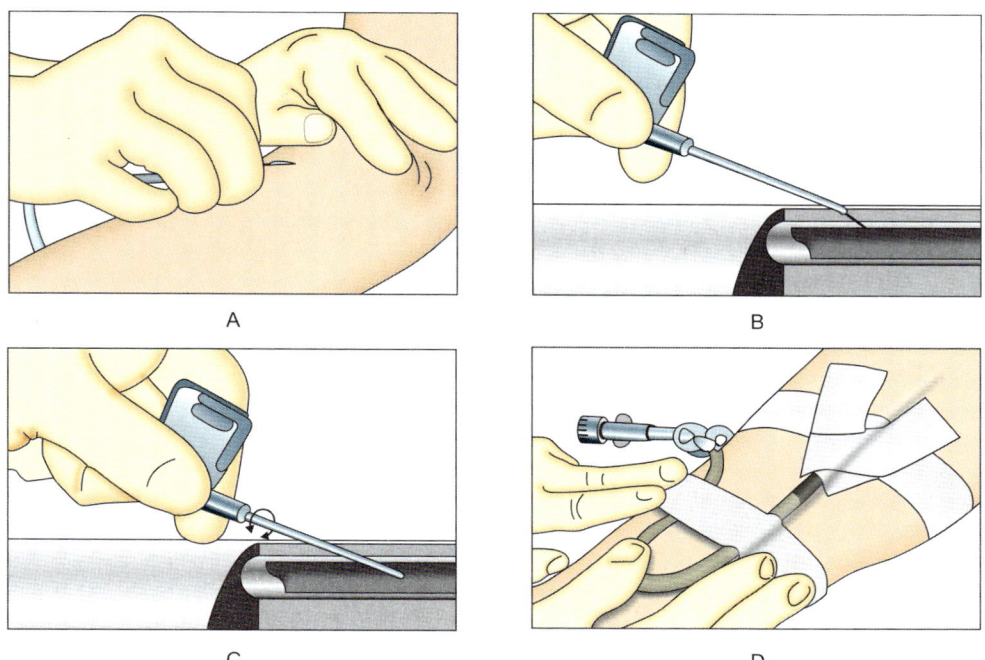

Fig. 7.1A to D: Technique of cannulation and position site or placement

5. Remove needle at the same or angle similar to angle to insertion, and never apply pressure before needle is completely out.

Cannulation of AVGs

Grafts generally should not be cannulated for at least 2 weeks after placement and not until swelling has subsided so that palpation of the course of the graft can be performed. The composite PU graft should not be cannulated for at least 24 hours after placement and not until swelling has subsided so that palpation of the course of the graft can be performed. Rotation of cannulation sites is needed to avoid pseudoaneurysm formation.

PREVENTION AND TREATMENT OF CATHETER AND PORT COMPLICATIONS

Catheters and ports should be evaluated when they become dysfunctional. Dysfunction is defined as failure to attain and maintain an extracorporeal blood flow of 300 ml/min or greater at a pre-pump arterial pressure more negative than 250 mm Hg.

Complicatns of Vascular Access

1. Infection
2. Catheter clotting
3. Central vein thrombosis or stricture
4. Stenosis or thrombosis
5. Ischemia of the hand
6. Aneurysm

Signs of Access Dysfunction

Methods that should be used to treat a dysfunctional or nonfunctional catheter or port include:

1. Repositioning of a mal-positioned catheter
2. Thrombolytics, using either an intraluminal lytic, intradialytic lock protocol, or an intracatheter thrombolytic infusion or interdialytic lock
3. Catheter exchange with sheath disruption, when appropriate

Treatment of an infected HD catheter or port should be based on the type and extent of infection.

Chapter 8

Guidelines, Instruction and Management of Risk Factors

ANTICOAGULATION/HEPARINIZATION

Purpose

To prevent clotting in the extracorporeal circuit during hemodialysis, anticoagulation is mandatory.

Scope

Effective anticoagulation increases dialyzer reuse rate, maintained efficacy and allows un-interrupted four hours dialysis session.

Procedure

In patients without elevated bleeding risk low-dose, unfractionated heparin or LMWH can be used to prevent clotting of the extracorporal system during hemodialysis. Because of proven safety, equal efficacy, and easy handling, the use of LMWHs is to be preferred over unfractionated heparin. Other benefits of LMWH are an improved lipid profile, less hyperkalemia and less blood loss.

Unfractionated Heparin

Unfractionated heparin binds to the heparin-binding site of antithrombin-III (AT-III). This induces conformational changes of AT-III resulting in the transition of AT-III from a slow into a rapid inactivator of clotting factors such as factor Xa and to a lesser extent XIIa, XIa, and IXa.

At present, routine anticoagulation with heparin is performed with low-dose heparin. Heparin is given by loading dose (approximately 50 IU/kg), followed by continuous infusion (800–1500 IU/h).

The efficacy of heparin treatment is evaluated by measurement of the activated partial thromboplastin time or the whole-blood clotting time. A prolongation of the APTT or whole-blood clotting time to 150% of their pre-dialysis values is recommended.

In case of overdosing or active bleeding after heparin administration, the effect of unfractionated heparin can be counteracted by the intravenous administration of protamine (1 mg protamine neutralizes 90–115 USP U heparin.

LMWHs

LMWHs are depolymerized fractions of heparin, and consist of smaller units. LMWHs are effective inhibitors of factor Xa. LMWHs not only are smaller but also less negatively charged. This results in reduced non-specific binding to plasma proteins and improved bioavailability.

A single bolus injection is usually suffice to avoid clotting of the extracorporal system. Additional LMWH (as a bolus or continuous infusion) is needed when the length of the dialysis sessions exceeds 4 h.

- Prevention of clotting in the HD patient with elevated bleeding risk

In patients with increased bleeding risks such as the phase immediately before and after surgery or in case of gastrointestinal blood loss, systemic anticoagulation should be avoided. Heparin free dailysis should be done.

Steps for heparin free dialysis are as follows:

1. No use of heparin during priming and during dailysis.
2. Remove all air from the dialyzer during the priming operation.
3. Regular saline flushing (flushed with saline 0.9% (100–300 ml every 30 min).
4. Absolute prevention of air introduction in the extracorporal circuit during dialysis.
5. A high blood flow rate from the beginning of treatment.
6. Prophylactically changing the dialyzer and blood lines.

Clotting of the dialyzer depends on the blood flow rate, heparinization, clotting parameters and HB level of patient. Frequent clotting decreases the efficacy of a dialyzer and makes it unsuitable for further use. Frequent changing of dialyzers impose huge financial burden on the patients. To avoid it dialyzer is reused.

When dialyzers are reused, it is reprocessed following the Association for the Advancement of Medical Instrumentation (AAMI) Standards and Recommended Practices for reuse of hemodialyzers.

Dialyzers intended for reuse have a blood compartment volume not less than 80% of the original measured volume or a urea (or ionic) clearance not less than 90% of the original measured clearance.

Steps of Dialyser Reprocessing

1. Rinsing and reverse ultrafiltration
2. Cleaning
3. Test of dialyzer performance: Pressure leak, FBV
4. Disinfection/sterilization
5. Documentation/labeling
6. Storage

Reuse Procedure for Hollow Fiber Dialysers

1. After closing the dialysis take the dialyser and tubing's to the cleaning place as soon as possible. (If delayed the blood will clot in the fibers and the dialyser will not reusable.)
2. Rinse the dialyser with flow of water from the venous end to the arterial end.
3. Rinse till the return flow of water from the dialyser is clear.
4. Reverse the flow of water from arterial end to venous end.
5. Disconnect the dialyser from the tap.
6. Close the outlet with a rubber cap.
7. Fill the dialysate compartment with hydrogen peroxide solution (2%)
8. Close the inlet with a rubber cap.
9. Leave the blood inlet and outlet ends open.
10. Keep the dialyser with hydrogen peroxide for a minimum of 30 minutes.
11. Open the inlet and outlet and empty the dialysate compartment.
12. Connect the RO water to the compartment and wash out the dissolved clots.
13. Check the fiber bundle volume. If the volume lost is more than 25%, discard the dialyser.
14. Lose the outlets and fill both the compartments with 4% formaldehyde/3% renaline.
15. Close the inlet and the outlet with caps.
16. Arrange them neatly and store then in the shelves and boxes provided.

Guidelines Instruction for Heparin Injection during Hemodialysis

Ensure that client does not have any history of (use only the 25.000 units/vial):

1. Bleeding piles/rectal bleeding
2. Excessive bleeding/vagina
3. Hemoptysis
4. Hematemesis

5. ICH
6. Liver disease/low platelets/recent surgery
7. Heamarthrosis
8. Hypertension (blood pressure above 150/80)
9. History of fall, injury
10. In clients on heparin infusion or on low molecular weight heparin, avoid heparin during dialysis (usually clients of cardiology and ICU clients)
11. In clients without bleeding tendency injection heparin 10, 000 unit diluted in 25 ml N/S is used. Use 5 ml from prepared mixture for injecting in circulation. Another 5 ml is given as bolus dose, 2.2 ml/hourly setting is done.

The machine is set in order that half an hour before termination of hemodialysis the heparin infusion stops the automatically.

Risk Factors of Hemodialysis (Dialysis instructions for AKD unit by Doctors)

- Explain the client and relatives that high blood pressure can cause life threatening complications like heart failure and stroke
- If heparin is also given it may lead to intra-cerebral hemorrhage (with death rate > 80%), retinal bleeding (lead to blindness) and intractable bleeding from any side.
- Good number of dialysis clients loses their life every year because of related complications

Clients Care Guidelines for Prevention of Transmission of Hepatitis "B"

1. All clients with hepatitis B infection (HbsAg positive) require special infection control precautions to prevent the spread of hepatitis B to other clients and associates
2. Staffs shall follow the guidelines and all clients shall be screened for hepatitis B prior to first dialysis treatment.
3. All clients shall be given hepatitis B vaccination monthly 3 doses and 6 monthly last dose be given and recorded

4. When changing care from HbsAg positive clients to HbsAg negative clients, gowns and face shield must be removed.

Infection Control in AKD Unit

1. To prevent or minimize the risk of infectious disease transmission among clients and staff.
2. Universal precautions shall be followed when providing care to all clients
3. Eating and drinking shall be confined to designated areas, outside eatables not allowed.
4. Suspected or known exposure to or acquisition of a communicable disease shall be brought to the notice of authority. All needle sticks shall be reported the same.
5. Personal protective equipment shall be worn for initiating and discontinuing hemodialysis and any time exposure to body fluids is anticipated. If clothing becomes soiled by blood and/or body fluids, it shall be changes immediately.
6. During the dialysis gloves shall be worn when touching or manipulating the client's fistula, shunt or intravenous catheter IV tubing, or any client's body fluids such as vomit, stool, urine, blood. gloves should be worn when touching the dialysis machine such as knobs, buttons, tubing, clamps, changing transducers or cleaning the machine.
7. Hand washing shall be performed before and after each client contact and after removal of gloves.
8. All cuts and lacerations shall be covered with a waterproof dressing.
9. Blood and other specimens fluids shall be handled with care using universal precautions.
10. Linen shall be handled appropriately.
11. Splashing, spilling or dripping of body fluids can become environmentally contaminated.

Nursing Intervention for Risk Reduction

1. Do not reprocess equipment in close proximity to clients
2. Select manufactures appropriate methods for sterilization of equipment
3. Use single—use disposable items as appropriate
4. Use sterile insertion trays separate for each client
5. Avoid multidose vials
6. Avoid splashing and spraying
7. Dispose off all lines and filters in hospital red biohazard infections waste bags and containers
8. Clean exterior of machine if obvious soiling occurs during dialysis
9. Prevent reflux of blood into monitoring systems
10. Observe for blood leaks
11. Filters that are reusable for 6 months should be disinfected when the machine is disinfected
12. Solutions can cause infections such as contaminated water source, contaminated dialysis fluid, contaminated blood lines and monitoring equipment, contaminated infusion system, contaminated venous pressure gauge
13. Prepare and use solutions aseptically and in a timely manner. Monitor viable microbial counts every month (it should not exceed 200 ml). Samples are collected quarterly with all results to be filled in Dialysis unit, samples are collected from every batch). Use aseptic technique during connecting/disconnecting procedure. Drain dialysate fluid directly into sewer system.
14. Infection control precautions such as all machines shall be given water rinse daily after talking clients. Every sunday all the machines shall be given sodium hypochlorite disinfection and Rena clean disinfection and kept over night. External cleaning of the machine is done daily either bacillocid or bacillol 25. Before taking clients machine are given RO water rinsing for 15 months and hot water rinse. Pressure isolators or transducer filters shall be used to prevent blood contamination. Venous pressure monitors. These isolators or filters shall be reused, 10 times. Dialyzers shall be reprocessed 10 times.
15. Between each client the external surfaces of the dialysis machine shall be disinfected bacillocid or bacillol 25
16. Citrosterile disinfection of each machine to be given on end of the day.
17. The internal fluid pathway of the dialysis machine shall be disinfected once every treatment day according to manufactures directions and regular cultures will be taken of the dialysate to ensure that the bacterila level in the dialysate is acceptable.
18. The disinfectant for dialysis machines shall have contact with parts of machine that are exposed to dialysis fluids, therefore the machine is to be removed for dialysis area, the drain line shall be removed from the drain and placed into a plastic bag for transportation. Clients known for HBsAg positive—a dedicated dialysis machine is to be used. If it is not possible the machine shall be decontaminated by cleaning all external surfaces with 1% lysoform solution prior to use on another clients.
19. A sterile hydrophobic transducer protector must be placed on each pressure fitting before connecting the pressure line to it. Otherwise, blood may enter the pressure monitor, causing disinfection problems and possible cross-contamination between clients. Replace the transducer protector between clients.
20. Always use an external transducer protector and utilize pressure alarm-capabilities as indicated in the manufactures' instruction. If the external transducer protector becomes wetted, replace it immediately and inspect it. If

fluid is visible on the side of the transducer protector that faces the machine, have qualified personnel open the machine and check for contamination after the treatment is completed. This check is to be included the internal pressure tubing set and pressure sensing port. Frequent bloodline pressure alarms or frequent adjusting of blood drip chamber levels may be an indicator.

Emergency ICU Client's Dialysis

Shifting client to ICU and back will be responsibility of the ICU/dialysis staff. The client should be accompanied by the duty nurse in charge of the client. She should remain with the client throughout the procedure. Hemodynamic monitoring using bedside, monitor to be jointly done by staff. ICU dialysis clients changes to be written in client's activity card by dialysis technician.

Clients Care Guidelines for Prevention of Transmission of Hepatitis "C"

Purpose: To avoid cross infection

Screening

1. Clients known to be HBSAg positive to HCV positive should be treated using dialysis unit precaution necessary.
2. Routine screening of dialysis clients for anti-HCV for purpose of infection control-monthly liver function tests (AST or ALT) shall be used as a screening method for HCV infection.

Guidelines for prevention of transmission of pulmonary tuberculosis: Responsibilities of staff involved-TB is highly infectious, airborne organism therefore appropriate room setting for ventilation and infection control policies and routine dialysis unit precautions followed. Screening, identification of client suspect TB should be evaluated. There are no restrictions on reuse of dialyzers of TB clients.

Chapter 9

Blood Transfusion

Purpose

To restore the blood volume.

Scope

Patients requiring blood and blood products during hemodialysis.

Responsibilities and Authorities

Consultant, CMO, RMO, dialysis staff nurse, blood bank staff.

Definition

Blood transfusion is the transmission of whole blood or its components such as blood cells and plasma from one person (donor) to other (recipient).

Procedure

Equipment

1. Sterile gloves
2. Blood infusion set
3. Blood/blood product as prescribed
4. Warmer

Method

Get the blood transfusion order from consultant doctor. Blood requisition form is filled. Relative is send for billing of cross-matching test to the billing counter. Then collect the blood sample from the patient and send it to lab for cross-matching and requisition of required blood to the blood bank.

Preparatory Phase

1. Inform the patient about the procedure, blood product to be given, approximate length of time and the out come of transfusion.
2. Obtain and record base line vital signs.
3. Obtain blood/blood product from blood bank and inspect for following: abnormal colour, cloudiness, clots and excess of air. Read instructions on the label regarding storage and inspection.
4. Check expiry date once the blood has reached the dialysis nursing unit, transfusion must be done within 30 minutes. Blood is checked for compatibility by RMO/CMO.
5. Verify patient's identification.
6. Ask the patient to state his full name and compare name with the wristband. If the patient is unable to state his name, verify infinity with an individual familiar with that patient.
7. Compare the name and the UHID number and wrist band with the bag transfusion form, medical order.
8. Confirm ABO and RH compatibility by comparing the bag label and medical record and or transfusion form.
9. Check bag label for expiry date.

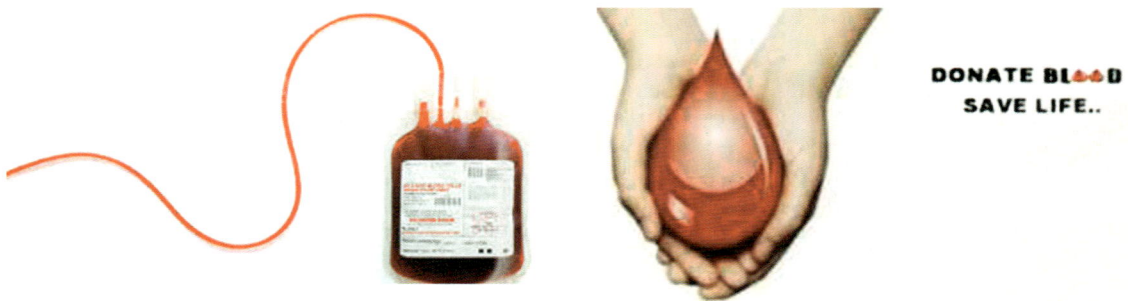

Fig. 9.1: Life is precious, blood gives life

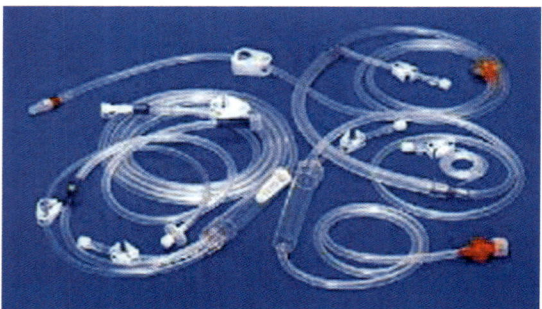

Fig. 9.2: HD unit tubings

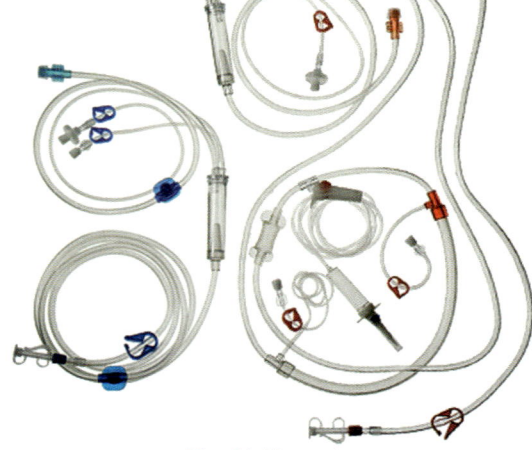

Blood tubing set

Fig. 9.4: Blood tubes

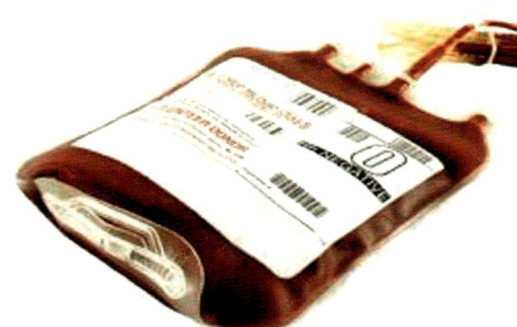

Blood pack

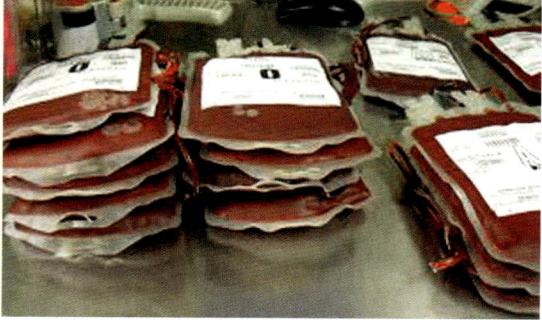

Fig. 9.3: Storage of blood packs

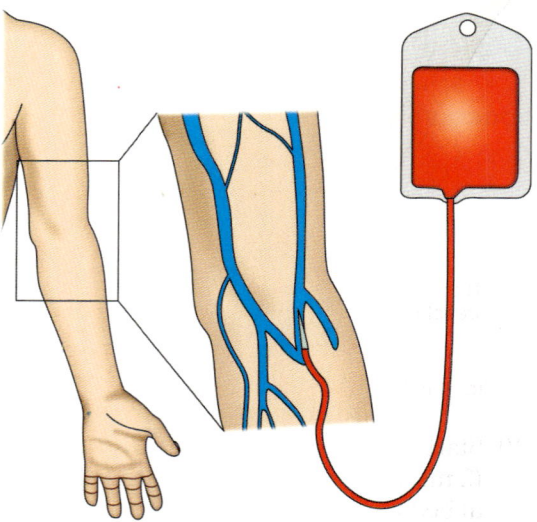

Fig. 9.5: Blood transfusion procedure

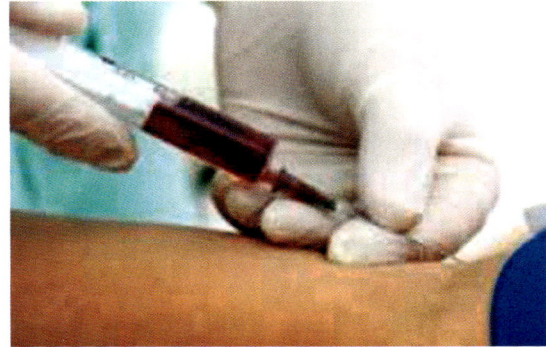

Fig. 9.6: Withdrawing blood

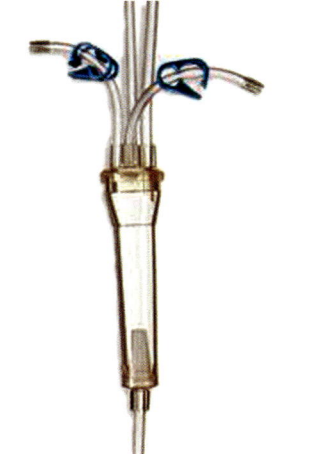

Fig. 9.7: IV set

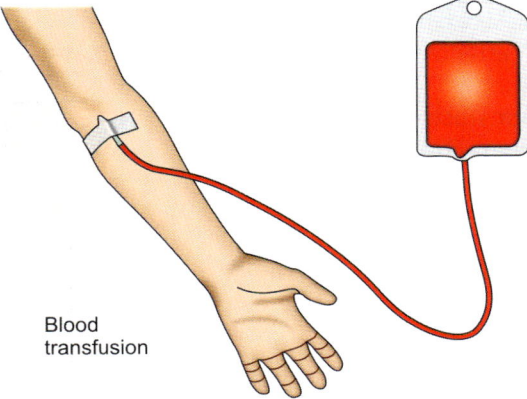

Blood transfusion

Fig. 9.8: Normal blood transfusion procedure

10. Start infusion slowly through saline line (2 ml/per minutes) 15–30 minutes remain at bedside. If there is no sign of an adverse reaction increase flow to the prescribed rate.

12. Observe the patient closely and check signs at least hourly until one hour after transfusion. Report signs and symptoms of adverse reactions to physicians immediately.

13. Record-time and name of the person starting and ending the transfusion. Name of the individual verifying patient ID. Clinical product identification number.

14. Product and volume infused.

15. Close the saline line after blood gets over from the bag.

Blood is one of the important constituents of our body fluid that is 7% of body weight.

Plasma constitutes 55%.

In order to maintain homeostasis in our body, if any components are reduced due to any condition, it should be replaced. Blood cells or platelets.

Blood transfusions are given to maintain hemoglobin level, to provide plasma-clotting factor, to help control in bleeding, to comb act infection or antibodies. It is indicated after surgery, trauma, hemorrhage, hemophilia, etc.

Selection of donor's time he should not have diseases of heart, liver, lungs, cancer, jaundice, tuberculosis, hepatitis, aids, allergies, pregnancy. Age from 18 to 65 and donors hemoglobin above 12%.

Blood transfusion begin slow first 15 minutes, if no reaction comes the flow can be increase and adjusted. Delay reaction can come even after several days. First 50 ml of transfusion anaphylactic reaction can appear. One ml 15 drops or 30 drops per minute as per order.

Observe for pre-masking BT reactions. Check label of the bag, HIV, Aids, HBC, expires date before the transfusion. Every two BT tubings are changed to decrease chances of bacteria.

Tridot-western blot-ELISA test done for HIV.

Blood Transfusion: Procedure

Standard Donation

- Veni puncture and blood withdrawal
- Standard precautions are used.
- Donors are place in a semi-recumbent position
- The skin over the antecunital fossa is carefully cleared with an antiseptic.
- Tourniquet is performed
- 450 ml blood withdrawal (within 15 minutes)
- Needle is removed
- Arm is told to hold straight up
- Firm pressure is applied with sterile gauze for 2–3 minutes.
- A firm bandage is then applied
- Patient kept in semi-recumbent position and made to sit when able.
- Food and fluids can be taken.
- No lifting heavy weight for several hours.
- Avoid smoking and drinking for 3 hours.
- Increase fluid intake for 2 days.
- Eat healthy meal for 2 weeks.

Transfusion of Packed Red Blood Cells (PRBCs) Pre-procedure

- Confirm that the transfusion has been prescribed.
- Check for patient's blood type and cross match
- Take consent
- Explain procedure s/s of transfusion reaction (itching, hives, swelling, shortness of breath, fever, chills)
- Take patient's vital
- Wash hands, wear gloves
- Use a 20 gauze or larger needle.

Procedure

- Obtain the PRBCs from the blood bank (1 unit at a time)
- Double check the lubes to make sure that the ABO group and Rh type agree with the compatibility record.
- Check patient's identification

- Check the blood for gas bubbles or unusual color or cloudiness (which indicate bacterial growth heterolysis).
- Make sure PRBC transfusion is initiated within 30 minutes after brought form blood bank.
- First 15 minutes run the transfusion slowly 5 ml/minute.
- Observe patient for adverse effects if no adverse effect increase flow rate.
- Monitor vitals regular interval
- If any adverse reaction stop BT
- Inform physical immediately
- Note administration time does not exceed 4 hours because of the risk of bacterial proliferation.
- Be alert for signs of circulatory overload, sepsis, febrile reaction, allergic reaction, and acute hemolytic reaction.
- Change blood tubing after every 2 units to decrease chances of bacterial contamination.

Post-Procedure

- Obtain vitals
- Dispose the materials properly
- Document the procedure
- Monitor patient for response to and effectiveness of the procedure.

Transfusion of Platelets/ Fresh-Frozen Plasma (FFP)

Same way points procedure.

Note: FFP requires ABO but not Rh compatibility. Platelets are not typically cross-matched fro ABO compatibility. Never add medications to blood or blood products.

PRBC—Never add medications to blood or blood products, if blood is too thick to run freely, NS may be added to the unit, if blood must be warmed, use an in-line blood warmer with a monitoring system.

Administration of blood and blood components requires knowledge of correct administration technique and possible complications.

What is Autologous Donation

A patient own blood may be collected for future transfusion. This method is useful in elective surgeries when need for transfusion is high. Preoperative donations are ideally collected 4–6 weeks before surgery. Iron supplements are prescribed during this period to prevent deplection of iron stores. Typically 1 unit of blood drawn each week. Advantage of this method is the prevention of viral infection from another person's blood; safe infusion, avoidance of complications, if blood is not required, it can be frozen until donor needs in future for up to 10 years. The blood is never returned to the general donor supply to be used for another person.

Disadvantages: It is expensive, takes time of uses resources inappropriately.

Intraoperative Blood Salvage

This transfusion method provides replacement for patient's who cannot donate blood before surgery. During a orthopedic or thoracic surgical procedure blood lost into a sterile cavity is suctioned into a cell-saver machine the whole blood washed often with NS filtered and then returned to the patient as an IV infusion. It cannot be stored.

Hemodilution

This method may be initiated before or after induction of anesthesia. About 1–2 units of blood are removed from the patient through a venous or arterial line and simultaneously replaced with a colloid or crystalloid solution. The blood obtained is then reinfused after surgery. Study that is more clinical is warned.

Blood Processing

Samples of the unit of blood are always taken immediately after donation, so that the blood can be typed and tested. Each donation is tested for antibodies HIV, HBC, HCV, human T-cell lymphotropic virus type 1 anti - HILV II /HbsAG, syphilis, and I.

A single unit of whole blood contains 450 ml of blood and 50 ml of an anticoagulant, which can be processed and disposed for administration. PRBCs are stored at 4°C with special preservatives they can be stored a safety up to 42 days before they must be discarded.

Plasma is immediately frozen to maintain the activity of the cloffing factors within, at last for 1 year if it remains frozen. Alternately, plasma can be further pooled and processed into blood derivatives, such as albumin, immunoglobulin. To treat hemophilia freeze dried concentrate of pooled fractnated human plasma used.

IN THERAPEUTIC APHERESIS

Blood is taken from patient and passed through a centrifuge, where a specific component is separated from the blood and removed the remaining blood is then returned to the patient. The entire system is closed so the bacterial contamination is low.

Purpose

Remove platelets, WBCs, RBC, plasma protein and remove circulating stem cells harvest.

Nursing Management for Transfusion Reaction

- Stop transfusion
- Maintain IV line with NS
- Maintain IV line it through new tubing administer at slow rate.
- Asses patient carefully
- Compare the vital signs with baseline (02 saturation) patient respiratory status, breath sounds mental status anxiety, confusion, chills, diaphoresis, jagular vein distension, back pain of urticaria,
- Notify physician.
- Notify blood bank
- Document reaction.

Assignment

- What are the potential causes of transfusion reaction?
- How are they manifested?
- What medical treatments would you anticipate?
- How should you educate the patient?
- What are the diseases that can be transmitted by BT, CHBS, HIV, CMV (cystomegalo-virus)
- GVHD (graft-verses-host-diseases) CJD, (Creutzfeldt-Jakob disease)
- What are the blood and blood components commonly used in transfusion therapy?
- Explain FFP (Fresh-Frozen plasma) with main complication of BT (fibrile nonhemolytic reaction, acute hemolytic reactions, allergic reaction, circulatory overload, bacterial contamination, and transfusion related acute lung injuring, delayed hemolytic reaction.

Chapter 10

Complications of Hemodialysis

Purpose

To minimize complication rate and mortality in the unit.

Scope

Hemodailysis is a dynamic procedure and can have numerous complications including life-threatening events like sudden death. Early recognition and prompt action of all complications are very important.

Responsibility

- Nephrologist
- Chief technician/nursing staff

Procedure

Complications during hemodialysis: complications are divided into 2 categories, common and uncommon.

Common complications are:

1. Hypotension
2. Muscle cramps
3. Nausea, vomiting
4. Chills and rigors
5. Headache back and Chest pain
6. Arrhythmias
7. Fistula failure
8. Fistula aneurysm and pseudo-aneurysm
9. Infections
10. Hypervolemia, hypovolemia
11. Bleeding at catheter site
12. Noninfectious catheter malfuction, obstruction dialysate leak.

Uncommon complications are:

1. Seizure
2. Hemodialysis disequilibrium
3. Anaphylactic reaction
4. Sudden death
5. Hemolysis
6. Air embolism

Management during Complication

- Reduce the pump speed.
- Raise the foot end.
- Give 100 to 150 ml of saline.
- Recheck the blood pressure and RBS
- If RBS is less than 70 mg, give 100 ml of 50% dextrose.
- If no response, return blood and fill saline in the tubes and keep it in recirculation
- Ask for ECG
- Call for RMO/nephrologist
- If no response from the patient start CPR
- Call anesthetist to secure airway
- Shift the patient into ICU

Initial Treatment for Common Complications

1. Hpotension
2. Reduce ultrafiltration rate
3. Reduce blood flow

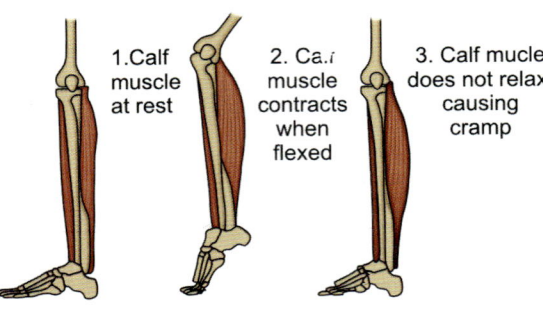

1.Calf muscle at rest   2. Ca./ muscle contracts when flexed   3. Calf mucle does not relax, causing cramp

Fig. 10.1: Muscle cramps

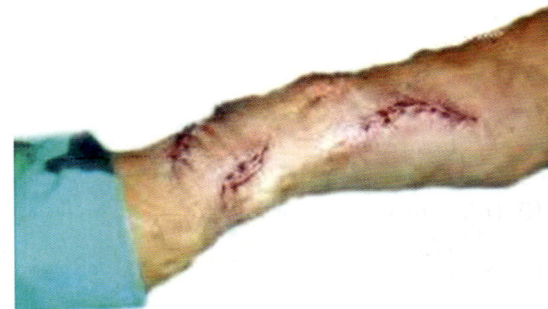

Fig. 10.4: Fistula complication malfunction, obstruction, dialysate leak

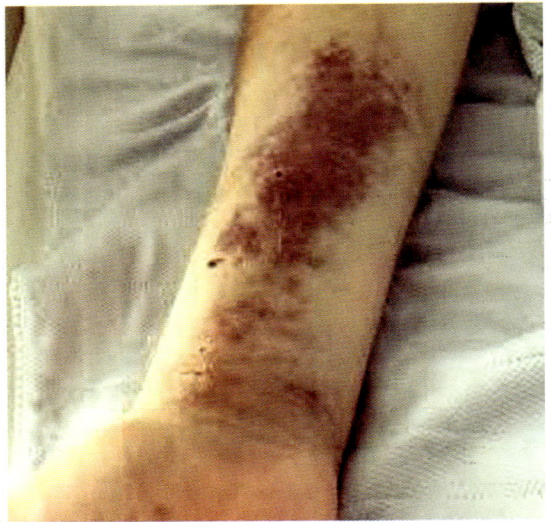

Fig. 10.2: Fistula failure bleeding at catheter site

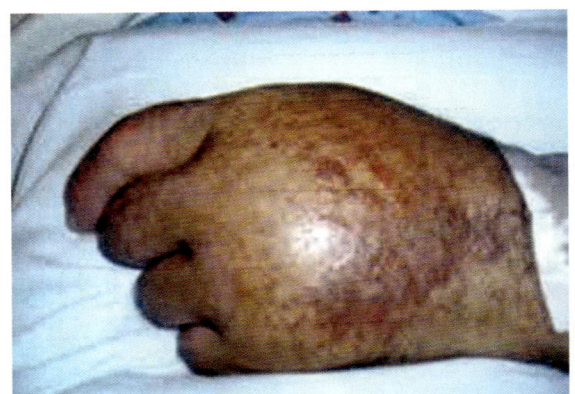

Fig. 10.5: Infection

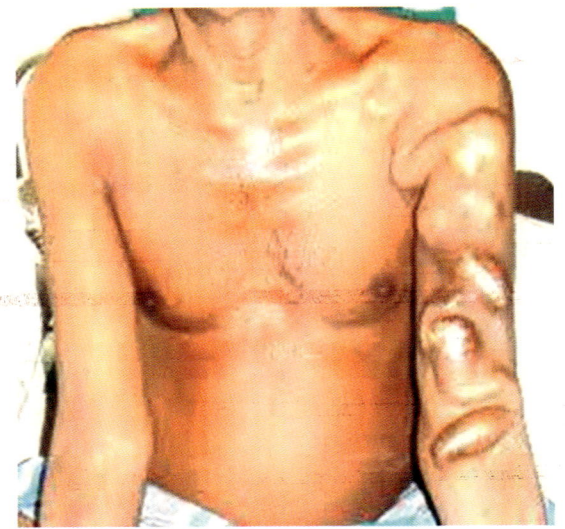

Fig. 10.3: Fistula complication hernia formation

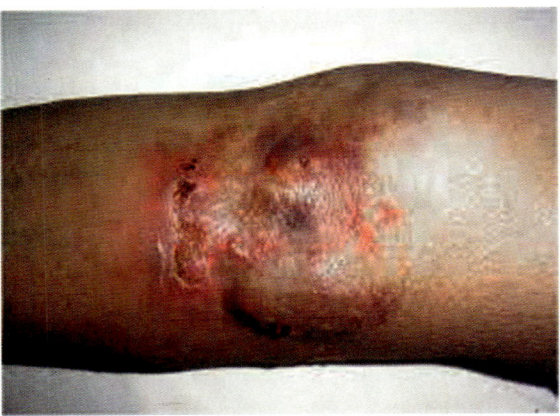

Fig. 10.6: Infection

4. Give 150–200 ml saline immediately
5. Raise the foot end
6. Get an ECG/ RBS
7. Inform RMO
8. Chills and rigors
9. Check temperature
10. Injection avil IV and hydrocortisone 100 mg IV
11. Paracetamol if temperature is more than 100° C
12. Nausea and vomiting
13. Check BP, if low give 150–200 saline
14. Injection emset 4.00 cc IV.
15. Injection patoprazole 40 cc IV

Muscle Cramps

1. Check BP, if low give 150–200 saline
2. Reduce ultrafiltration rate
3. Stretching exercise

Chapter 11

Diet during Hemodialysis

RESTRICTED DIET DURING HEMODIALYSIS

If you are receiving Hemodialysis treatments, your diet is an important part of your overall care. Getting the right amount of calories is important to your overall health and helps to give you energy to do the activities you enjoy.

The prescribed diet varies with severity of the disease and the type of maintenance treatment used. In the early stages, protein restrictions may be based on the glomerular filtration rate the protein intake must be adjusted to compensate for loss and catabolism of body protein. Calorie intake must be sufficient to permit activity without breakdown of tissue protein. Nutritional management in chronic renal failure is complex. Because of the multiplicity of factors to be considered in determining dietary modification for each individual, since diet is such an important part of disease management patient needs support of family, nurse, as well as dietitian. Food and fluids intake must be closely monitored and adjusted to the manifested needs. Total parenteral nutrition may also be used to maintain adequate nutrition for the critically ill patient.

Protein before you started dialysis; you may have been on a low-protein diet to limit the amount of waste products in your blood. Now that you have begun dialysis, your diet will include more protein. Getting the right amount of protein is important to your health and how well you feel. Your body needs the right amount of protein for building muscles, repairing tissues and fighting infections. Protein rich foods include fresh meats, poultry chicken, fish and other seafood, egg or egg white, small servings of dairy products, pulses. Some of these protein rich foods may also contain a lot of phosphorous, a mineral you may need to control in your diet.

Potassium is another important mineral found in food. Potassium helps your muscles and heart work properly. Too much or too little potassium in your blood can be dangerous. With hemodialysis, you will probably need to limit your intake of high potassium foods. The level of potassium in your blood will be checked every month, and your dietitian will help you plan a diet that will give you the right amount of potassium. Large amount of potassium are found in certain fruits and vegetables like bananas, melons, oranges, potatoes, tomatoes and some juices. Milk and milk products, dried beans and peas, most salt substitutes, protein rich foods such as meat, poultry and fish.

Sodium and fluids is a mineral found naturally in foods. It is found in large amounts in table salt such as seasoning garlic or onion salt, most canned foods and some frozen dinners, processed meats, salted snack foods like chips and crackers, dehydrated soups such as packed noodle soup, most restaurant and take out foods. Eating too much of sodium may make you thirsty and cause your body to hold onto more fluid. This can cause swelling or puffiness around eyes, hands or feet, fluid weight gain, shortness of breath, a rise in blood pressure, more work to your heart. Learn to flavor your foods with herbs and spices instead of table salt. Do not use salt substitutes containing potassium unless approved by your doctor.

Vitamins and minerals eating a wide variety of foods give your body the vitamins and minerals it needs each day. In addition to your good diet your doctor may order special vitamin and mineral supplements. Kidney disease and dialysis change the mounts of vitamins and minerals your body needs. In addition, your special diet may limit some

Dialysis Diet

Table 11.1: Dietary management: Two-week sample menu for hemodialysis patients (provides 80 gm of protein)

	Sunday	Monday	Tuesday	Wednesday
Breakfast	Scrambled eggs, 2 White toast, 1 slice Margarine, 1 tsp Cranberry juice, 4 oz Cofee/tea, 8 oz	Cheerios, 1/2 cup white Non-dairy creamer, 1/2 cup White toast, 1 slice Margarine, 1 tsp Coffee/tea, 8 oz	French toast, 2 slice, Eggs, 2+ White bread, 2 slices Margarine, 2 tsp Maple syrup, 4 tbsp Grape juice, 4 oz Coffee/tea, 8 oz	Cornflakes, 1/2 cup non-Non-dairy creamer, 1/2 cup Bagel, 1 Jam/jelly, 2 tsp or cream cheese, 2 tsp Grapefruit, 1 half Coffee/tea, 8 oz
Lunch	Sliced turkey sand-wich (1): Turkey, 3 oz Sourdough bread, 2 slices Mayonnaise, 1 tbsp. T cuttee, 1 leaf Tangerine, 1medium Regular/diet sprite, 4 oz	Hamburger (1): Lean beef patty, 3–4 oz on a hamburger bun Lettuce, 1 leaf Chopped onion, 1 tbsp Sliced mushrooms, 1/4 cups orange sherbet 3/4 cup iced tea, 4 oz	Grilled salmon, 3 oz Mexican pasta, 1 cup** Corn bread roll ,1 Margarine, 1 tsp Mixed green salad, 1/2 tup, oil and vinegar dressing: Salad/olive oil, 2 tsp, vinegar, 1 tsp., grapes, 15 medium regular/diet sprie, 4 oz	Tuna sandwich (1): Low sodium/water packed tuna, flaked, 4 oz. Mayonnaise, 1 tbsp, chopped onions, 1 tbsp, chopped celery, 1 tbsp, hard bread roll, 1 apple, 1 medium regular/ diet root beer, 4 oz
Dinner	Broiled garlic shrimp, 3 oz.* Rice, 1/2 cup Asparagus, 4 spears Dinner roll, 1 Margarine, 1 tsp Pineapple tidbits, 1/2 cup, Regular/diet root beer, 4 oz	Oven-baked chicken, 4 oz Mashed potatoes, 1/2 cup Margarine, 2 tsp, Caroots 1/2 cup, Applesauce 1/2 cup, Crystal light, 4 oz	Salisbury steak, 4 oz, with Slice mushrooms, 1/2 cup Chopped onions, 1/4 cup Noodles, 1/2 cup Dinner roll, 1 margarine 1 tsp. Green beans, 1/2 cup, Jell-O, 1/2 cup Lemonade, 4 oz	Baked pork chop, 3 oz Rice 1/2 cup, Steamed broccoli, 1/2 cup margarine 1 tsp. Canned apricots, 3 halves, Iced tea, 4 oz
Snack	Graham crakers, 2 squares, Canned pears 3 halves	Vnilla wafers, 6, Fruit cocktail, 1/2 cup	Baked apple with: sugar, 2 tsp Margarine, 2 tsp Cinnamon, 1 tsp	Chili wheat treats, 1/2 cup*

*Living well on dialysis   **Southwest cookbook   +Egg substitute/egg whites can be used in place of whole eggs

Importance of Diet Management: Figures 11.1 to 11.5 show restriction or adjustment of protein, sodium, potassium or fluid intake

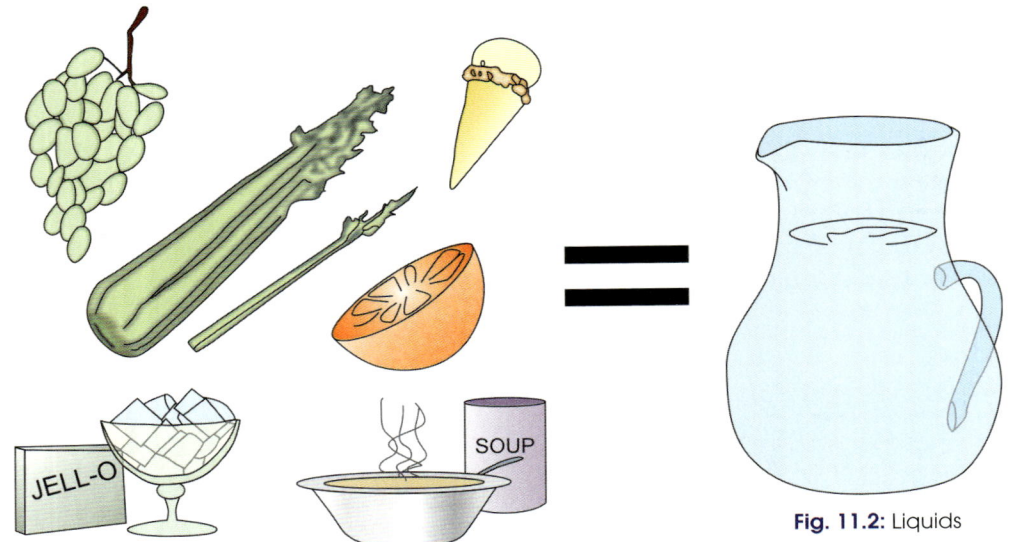

Fig. 11.1: Proteins

Fig. 11.2: Liquids

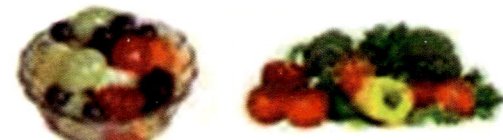

Low sodium diet

Low potassium diet

Low phosphorus diet

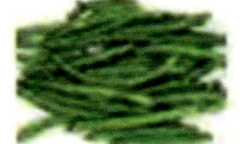 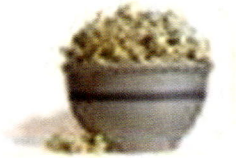

Fig. 11.4: Vegetables

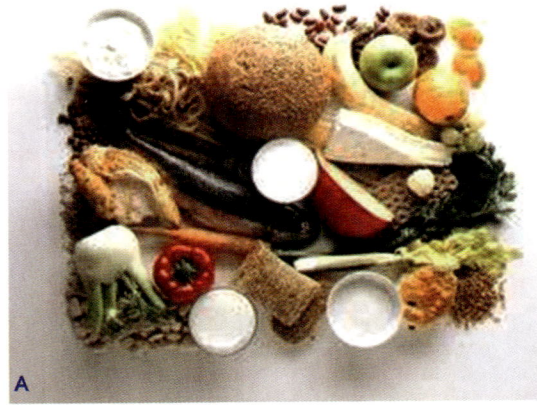

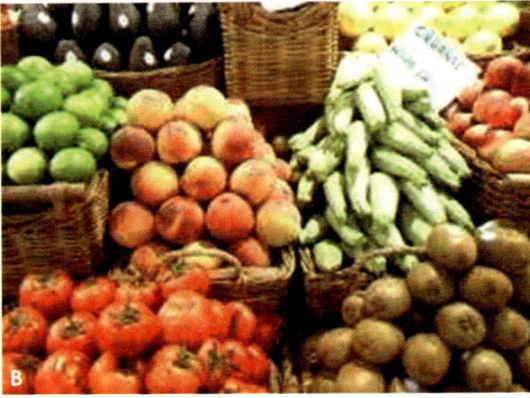

Fig. 11.3A and B: Vitamins and minerals

Which fruit is totally prohibited for a patient in dialysis?

- 7%
- 44%
- 45%
- 4%

■ Banana
■ Orange
□ Star-fruit or carambola
□ Papaya

Fig. 11.5: Amount of diet percentage to be avoided

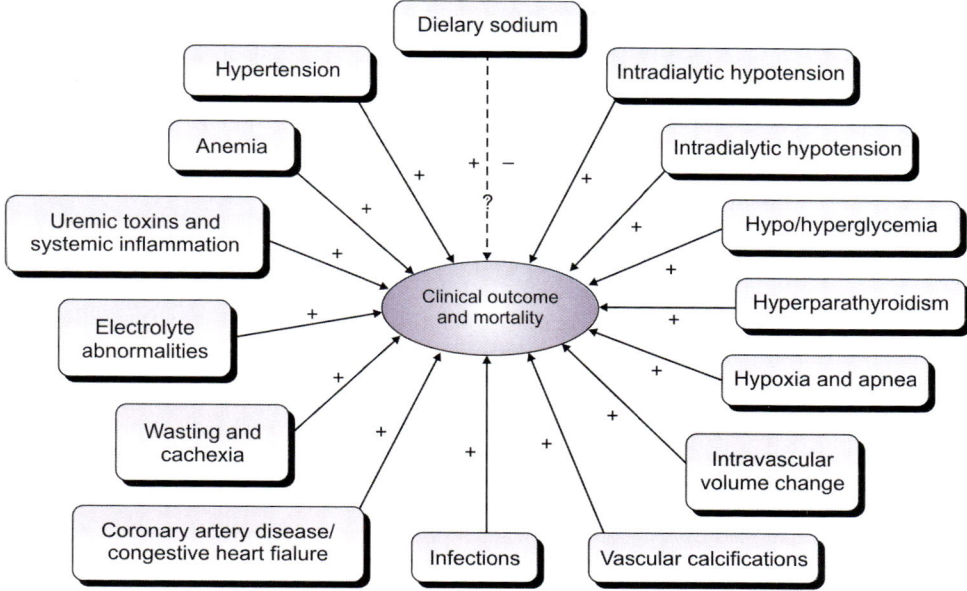

Fig. 11.6: Keep vigilance for complications of hemodialysis client

food groups that would provide important vitamins and minerals. Take only those supplements that are ordered by your doctor since certain vitamins and minerals can be harmful if you are on dialysis. In addition, check with your doctor before using any herbal remedies as some of these may be harmful for people with kidney disease.

Phosphorus is a mineral found in all foods. Large amount of phosphorus found in dairy products such as milk, cheese, yogurt, ice cream and pudding. Nuts and peanuts, dried beans and peas such as kidney beans, spilt peas, beverages such as cocoa, beer and dark cola drinks. Phosphorus addictives are in processed meats such as chicken refrigerated, bakery products and some beverages. Eating food high in phosphorus will raise the amount of phosphorus in blood. Dialysis cannot remove all of this phosphorus, when it is built up in your blood; calcium is pulled from the bones. Over time, your bones will become weaker and break easily. A high level of phosphorus in your blood may also cause calcium phosphorus crystals to build up in

your joints, muscles, skin, blood vessels and heart. These depositions may cause serious problems such as born pain, damage to the heart and other organs, poor blood circulation and skin ulcers. To keep blood phosphorus at safe levels, you will need to limit phosphorus rich foods and may need to take a type if medicine called phosphate binder. These binders are taken with your meats and snacks.

Calcium is a mineral that is important for building strong bones. However, foods that are good sources of calcium are also high in phosphorus. The best ways to prevent loss of calcium from your bones are to follow a diet that limits high phosphorus food and to take phosphate binders. Your doctor may also prescribe a special form of vitamin D to help you keep calcium and phosphorus levels in balance and to prevent bone diseases. Do not take over the counter vitamin D unless recommended by your kidney doctor.

Important Points

1. Your doctor will determine what your ideal body weight should be. Hence weigh

yourself each day in the morning and keep him informed about any fluctuation in your body weight.

2. If you are loosing too much weight, ask your doctor how to add extra calories to your diet.

3. If you are slowly gaining too much weight, ask for suggestions on safely reducing your daily calorie intake and increasing your activity level.

4. If you gain weight rapidly, speak to your doctor and dietitian. A sudden increase in weight, along with swelling, shortness of breath and a rise in your blood pressure may be a sign that you have too much fluid in your body.

Other common facts about the food and nutrition of a common man who may not be under dialysis can follow:

Relation of nutrition and health is how the food eaten and how the body uses it. Food is made up of different nutrients need for health and growth. Nutrition deals with the way in which human body receives and uses all the substance and materials necessary for growth, development, repair and how the body is kept in good condition.

The food eaten that is digested and broken into simple substances then they are absorbed into the blood stream and carried to the liver where it is stored and sent out to different parts of the body as per requirement.

Some are used to supply the body with heat and energy where as others for building and repair of the tissues. Some protect the body from disease and some control the chemical changes that takes place in the body. So all the nutrient needed by the body should be available in the food we consume.

There are many kinds of food combination to make the balance diet compete. No food by itself has all the nutrients it has to be teamed with other nutrients and we need them in varying amounts, so there is relation to nutrition we take our health maintenance.

An adequate diet should contain liberal amounts of protein rich and protective foods. It should provide the dietary requirements that are essential in adequate amount and the quality of food consumed by different groups has a significance effect on the health.

There are foods that are animal origin, food of vegetable origin. There are foods that provide energy, other builds the body, other protect the body from harmful effect. The body is composed of protein, fat, carbohydrate, water and minerals.

Example below of a man weighing 65 kg

Protein	11 kg	17%
Fat	9 kg	13.8%
CHO	1 kg	1.5%
Water	40 kg	61.6%
Minerals	4 kg	61%

CHO are essentials for the oxidation of fats and are part of tissue constituents. They are required for the proper functioning of liver, heart and muscle contraction. Excess CHO are converted to fat and stored, in balanced diet about 50–60% of energy supplied by it

Age group optimal level of CHO calculated as total calories as follows:

Infant	40–50%
Pre-schooled	40–60%
Older children	50–70%
Adolescents	50–70%
Adult	50–70%
Expectant and nursing mothers	40–60%

Metabolism of CHO-glucose, galactose and fructose absorbed in the intestines pass through the portal circulation in the liver. There it is converted into glycogen and part of it goes into the general circulation and to the various tissues for oxidization and used as energy. A small part of it stored in liver and muscle as glucogen and some portion of it is converted into fat and stored into the adipose tissue.

Proteins are found in all living cells both plants and animals. They are important nutrients. They are broken down into amino acid. Body can make 12 amino acids and 8 are known to be essential which come from the food. Digestion of protein takes place into the stomach, intestines. The amino acids are absorbed in the small intestines and enter into the blood circulation through the portal vein. Its functions are to replace the daily loss of body protein, formation of tissue during growth, formation of enzymes and certain hormones, growth of the fetus in pregnancy and for the production of milk during lactation due to its deficiency kwashiorkor, nutritional marasmus results.

Vitamins are organic compounds which body required in small amount for growth and maintenance of good health. Prolong deficiency causes illness, e.g. night blindness, anemia, scurvy, etc.

Signs of Poor Nutrition

1. Appearance is listless, apathetic, emancipated, wasted, underweight, posture is sagging shoulders, sunken chest, humped back, muscles poor tone, tender, under developed, inability to walk properly.
2. Attention deficit
3. Irritable, confused
4. Burning and tingling of hands and feet's
5. Weakness and tenderness of muscle or loss of ankle and knee reflexes. Anorexia, indigestion, constipation and diarrhea, liver or spleen enlargement, easily fatigued, no energy.
6. Falls asleep easily, looks tired, apathetic, dull, brittle, dry, thin hair, skin rough, scaly, pale, easily bruised, delayed wound healing, lips fissures at the corner, stomach gums spongy bleed easily, tongue beefy, bitots spots, thyroid enlargement, edema, bowlegs, knock knees, etc.

7. Financial status—limited amount of money, is to be inadequate food to prevent hunger is difficult to meet nutritional needs
8. Geographical location affects the availability of many fresh food items, meats and sea foods, culture, child rearing practices, eating utensils, mealtimes, eating food pattern/concerning new flavoring and cooking system, religion, social circumstances, appropriate social contacts, age, poor food hygiene, excessive exposure to sun, not eating variety of foods, too much sugar, more salty, drink alcohol, eat saturated fat, adding food addictives.
9. Good health is based on good nutrition; poor nutrition causes illness of the body and mind. Prolonged severe deficiency can causes bony an teeth disorders. Causes anemia, apathy.
10. Learn new therapeutic dietary regimen, new diet.
11. Role of food in diet is vital, food is ingested, digested, absorbed, transported and used nutrition to maintain circulation, respiration, muscle tone, body temperature and other basal energy requirements and fuel is provided daily by it.
12. Food patterns, duration of meal, kind of food eaten, amount of food eaten, items, time likes and dislikes, intolerance, appetite, monmey available for food purchasing, preparation, storage, al these aspects are important to determine.
13. Some people completely exclude some type of foods entirely, certain food may be inappropriate needs reasonably dietary modification food preferences and eating habits, snacks play a role in food intake, each human being is unique in specific nutritional requirements for optimal function. It is related to tests, texture, flavor preferences. Acceptable and unacceptable foods. Media influence food related behaviour, educate public concerning can alter food intake. Nutrients

and foods can alter medication absorption and medication can alter nutrition absorption, metabolic and excretion.

14. Alter nutrition less o more than body requirements, inability of ingest sufficient nutrition impaired swallowing, breast feeding, dysfunctional eating pattern, lack of physical activity, lack of exercises, eating due to response to stress or emotional trauma, lack of food, lack of interest in food, lack of information, misinformation or misconception, insufficient digestion, weak mastication or swallowing.

Chapter 12

Organ Donation and Kidney Transplantation

Organ Donation

To prolong the life span of kidney failure patients and prevent mortality—**Save lives through organ donation**—remember, lakhs of patients are dying because there are not enough donors. Be the change, pledge your organs.

Brain death is irreversible loss of all brain functions, usually due to serious head injury or stroke. After brain death is declared, 34 vital organs and tissues can be retrieved using artificial support to keep the blood supply going. In normal or cardiac death, heart stops beating, cutting off blood supply to organs. Skin and cornea can be retrieved; families need to contact a doctor immediately to initiate the organ donation process.

Organ donation is important as one body can give a new lease of life to those suffering from blindness, lung, liver, stomach and kidney disorders, heart ailments, pancreatic infections and bone problems. It can be donated too. In fact, cadaver donation is the best gift one can give to others. Organ donation does not leave the body disfigured. Organs are removed with the greatest care and dignity by a team of specially trained surgeons. The transplantation of human organ Act and Rules, as amended from time to time, recognizes the concept of brain death and gives a legal sanction for diagnosis of brain death and deceased organ donation.

Jewish view on organ donation: Modern technology has made it possible to transplant organs like heart, kidney, cornea, lung and liver from one human being to another, to save or enhance the quality of life of patient who suffers organ damage. What could be more altruistic than the gift of life? Once you are dead, your body need not go waste. The dead body is the shell of a living image of God. Being willing to donate organ from our own bodies would be great example of selfless sacrifice for another. One time organ donation was prohibited in Jewish, today that is not the case. Let us declare in one voice, that I would like to help someone to live even after my death.

Give life after death: It is tragic that the lack of cultural awareness and reliable medical infrastructure keeps organ donations low. India 0.16/million population compared to Americans 26 and Spains 35. It is a sensitive subject. Harvesting organs from a dead body may appear a dead body logical from a scientific point of view. Nevertheless, human beings are not creatures of logic alone. True extracting healthy organs from a dead body might help save lives. However, this decision can only done by individual alone. For even in death the human body is a representation of the person someone child, father, mother or husband or wife. Mutilating the dead body for its organs could be perceived as and in many cases is an insult to the human emotions that bind the decreased person with his loved ones. These sentiments are also informed by religions beliefs that treat the human body as a sacred vessel. Such resistance in matter of faith. Islam prohibits defilement of the body. Hinduism prescribes a set of ritual to help the soul of the decreased journey to the next life.

Modern medicine can deliver miracles via transplant surgery. The basic magic is that in death, a human being can extend that life of up to 50 other human beings. After patient is declared brain dead doctor can harvest 37 different organ and tissues to help others, a blind person can see again, a child born with a hole in heart could laugh.

Health and happiness: The secret of health for both mind and body is not to mourn for the past, not to worry about the future, or not to anticipate troubles, but to live in the present moment wisely and earnestly. Health is a state of complete harmony of the body mind and spirit. When one is free from physical disabilities and mental distractions, the gates of the soul open. If you have health, you probably will be happy and if you have health and happiness, you have all the wealth you need, even if it is not all you want.

Kidney Transplantation

The development of donor selection by tissue typing and the steady progress that has been made in managing the rejection process, have resulted in an increase in the number of kidney transplants.

An advantage of a kidney transplant for the person who has severe renal failure is the discontinuation of the demanding dialysis schedule, considerable time is saved and patient becomes more productive. Dietary restrictions are lifted and constraint of activity is slight. The patient must be aware of the possible adverse effects as well as the benefits of transplantation prior to deciding the mode of treatment. Transplantation requires major surgery and a life-long dependency on immunosuppressive drugs. Rejection of the transplant necessitates return to dialysis and consideration for re-transplantation.

Transplant Procedure

The donor's kidney is placed in the recipient's iliac fossa, usually on the side opposite to that from which it was taken that is a left donor kidney is placed in the recipients right iliac fossa. Its renal artery may be anastomosed to the host's hypogastric artery, and the renal vein of the graft is anastomosed to the common or external iliac vein. The ureter is implanted in the recipient's bladder via a sub-mucosal tunnel, the latter prevents urinary reflux. A J-stent may be inserted into the transplanted kidneys ureter to prevent obstruction. It will normally be removed by cystoscopy after three months.

The patients own kidneys are removed if there is recurrent infection or uncontrolled hypertension. Polycystic kidneys may need to be removed to provide room for the graft.

The patient is instructed to keep a daily record of his weight, fluid amount and medication taken. Suggestions are made as to how he may protect himself as much as possible from infection.

Donate a patch of life in severe burn cases; there is high mortality and morbidity due to infection and dehydration. They also suffer severe pain. Much of this can be prevented if they get human skin to cover the burn area, patient start generating their own skin. Thus, human skin is a lifesaver for such patient skin harvesting is a simple procedure, within 6 hours of death, relatives can call helpline doctors and a technician will arrive within 45 minutes with special instrument skin can be taken. It is harvested from the legs, thighs and back. Only an eight of the thickness of the skin is removed and there is no bleeding after that the body is bandaged and no disfigurement is noticeable.

The skin is preserved in glycerol solution and transported to the skin bank. After

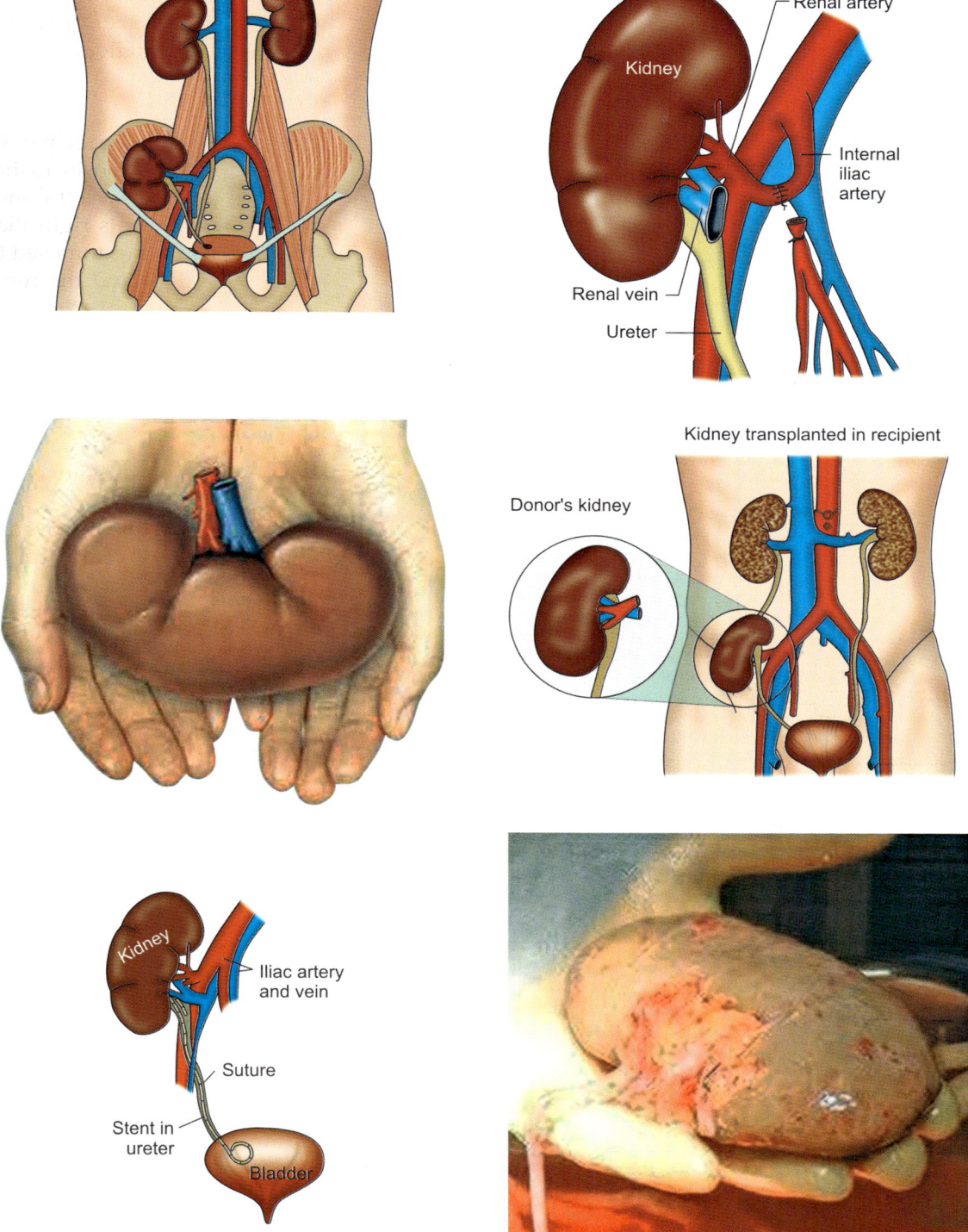

Fig. 12.1: Surgically removal and kidney transplant technique

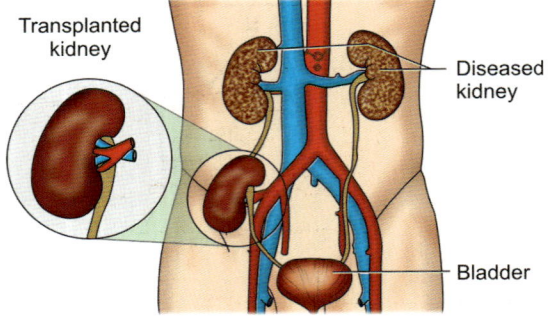

Transplanted kidney

Diseased kidney

Bladder

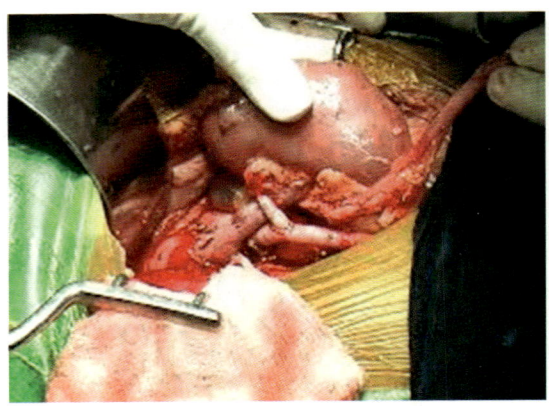

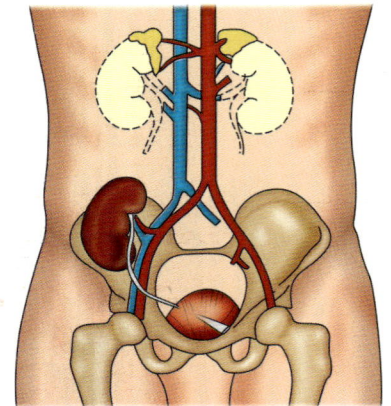

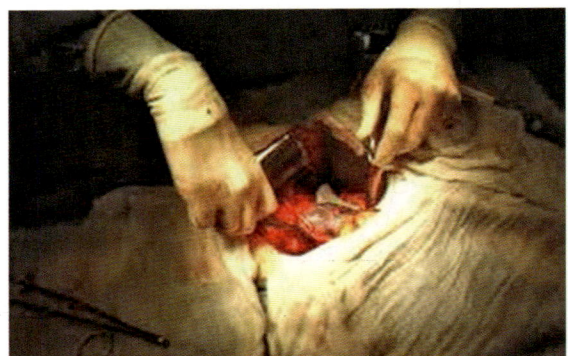

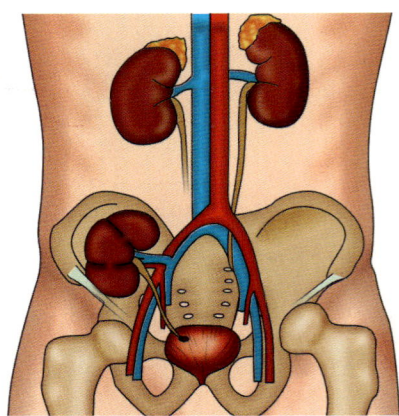

Fig. 12.2: Different view and angle of surgically removal and transplant procedure

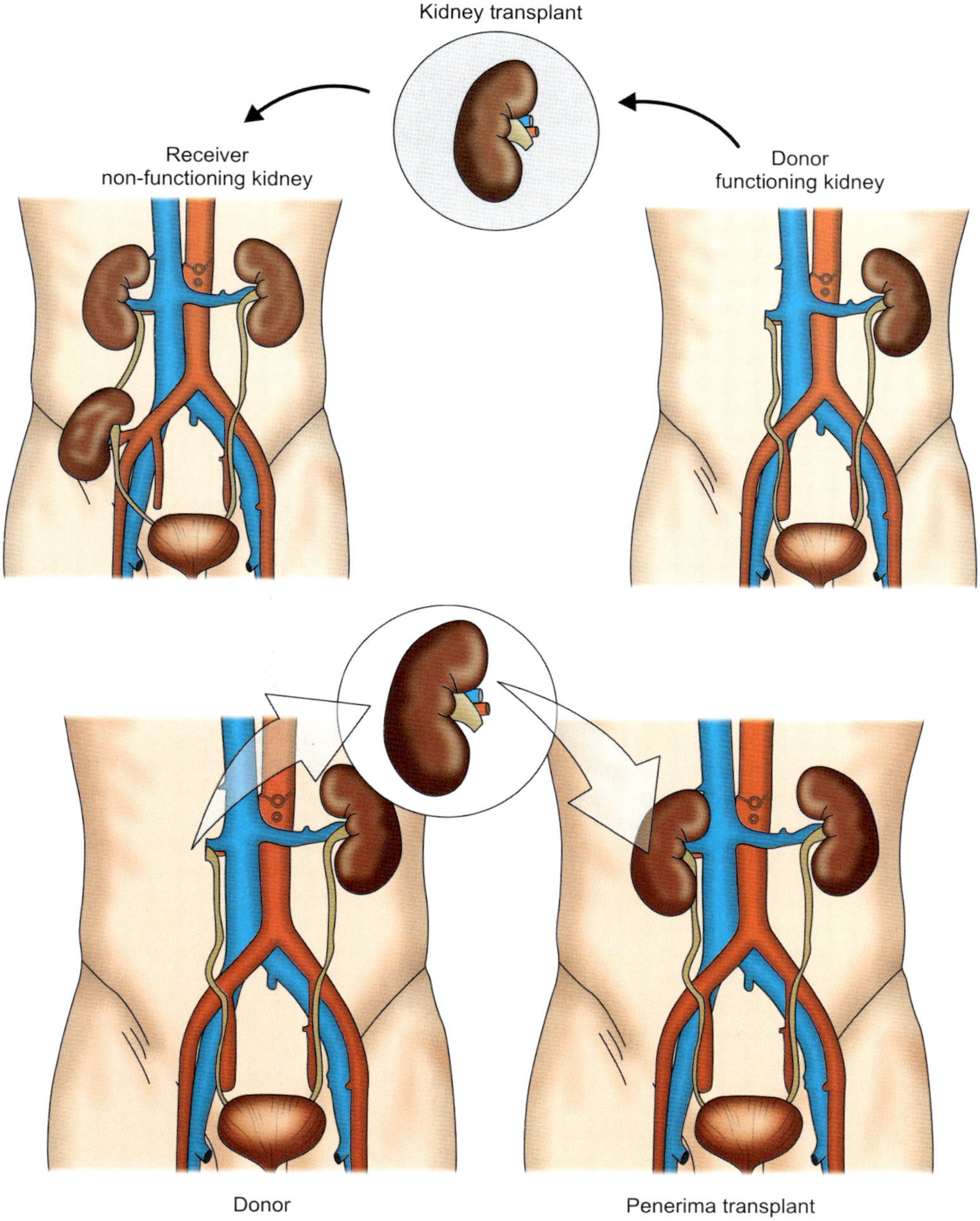

Fig. 12.3: Kidney transplant procedure before and after

processing, it is stored in a special cold room. It can be preserved for 5 years. A blood sample is also drawn to check for HIV infection. Australian antigen and septicemia. No donor-recipient, blood or color matching is required. Consent and death certificate is needful

Skin donation is lagging, with donor reluctant to part with it.

Donation of skin: Skin grafting is the only option to reconstruct badly burnt body parts. Cultural stigma continues to discourage people. Raw skin takes a minimum of 14–21 days to heal and donated skin would give temporary cover for a week at least. The body will eventually reject the donated skin. But until the new skin grows we can use the donated skin to buy time. Education awareness is must.

Organ donation: The only hope for patients suffering from organ failure is transplantation. However, there is a universal shortage of donors, largely due to lack of information, misconception and ignorance. India where fear of violating the sanctity of the decreased and other myths contribute too keeping donor number low

Do not save for after life: For some the fear of donating is real as fear of death. The biggest myth is the belief in life after death. Many people think if they donate an organ, they will have to survive without it in their after life.

Donors do not pay: Ignorance is a big hurdle. Common fears include burdening the family with the expense of donating ones organ, or that ones organs might not be healthy enough for harvesting. We have to reiterate that donors are not charged anything and it's actually the doctors call whether an organ is healthy or not.

It is myth that if people have weak eyes, they cannot donate. If you have a healthy cornea: The black part of the eye—you can donate even if you have a weak retina. At the time of death, the entire eyeball is taken out by ultimately only the cornea is used.

No personality change: Indians feel more strongly that transplants would affect their behaviour. Recipients preferred to get an organ, DNA transplant or blood transfusion from a donor whose personality matched theirs. It is surprising since BT are so common, we expected people might think they have very little effect.

Bodies are not disfigured: People are also afraid that cadaveric donation leaves the body disfigured. But sectors actually take care to prevent that the human body is sacred, organ removal will not disfigure or alter the appearance of the body nor it will interferes with customary funeral or burial arrangements. After surgery, the body is stitched up very carefully.

Life sacred: The quality of care will not change, regardless of your decision to donate. The doctors involved in saving your life are entirely different from the team involved in recovering organs and tissues. Believe in saving lives, not in myths

Sri Sri Ravi Shankar says: Donate your organs, it will earn you more *punya*. There can be no greater *karma* than offering every part of our body in the service of others. Come let us pledge ourselves to organ donation

Maulann Wahduddin Khan says some people are against organ donation, but its their personal opinion. We have to differentiate between personal opinion and the correct teaching of Islam. Organ donation is the noblest form of charity.

When did you pledge your organs?
(Interview)

Conscious effort to contribute to the huge requirements for vital organs in India. So many people are suffering from kidney failure, end stage liver disease and other serious illness.

How did family react to the idea? They are supportive

Have you tried to encourage your teammates and others to pledge for organ donation

Aim is creating awareness about it.

Make conscious effort towards promoting the cause.

Surveys show that most people do not donate organs because of religious beliefs, what is your take?

What can give you more happiness and satisfaction that giving life to another individual even after death.

So many lives can be saved from one cadaver donation.

How the brain death established?

Brain death in India is determined by a series of clinical tests performed by 4 doctors-independently. They are not the part of there transplant team and are neurologists or neurosurgeon who have been certified by the state authority, the doctor talking care of the patient, as well as the medical head and the hospital.

Tests are conducted to rile out any other reasons that could be causing the brain not to function, such as medical conditions medication overdose, intoxication (alcohol) depressant drugs relaxants (neuromuscular blocking agents) or extreme cold. Death is indicated if the patient cannot breathe, without assistance, have neither pupil response to light nor response to pain.

An apnea test is performed to determine if the person can breathe on his own. Here, the doctor will disconnect the patient from the ventilator and check blood gas levels. A brain dead person will not breathe on his own and the carbon dioxide levels in his blood gas will be very high.

These tests have to be repeated by all 4 doctors after 6 hours to make a final declaration. Once brain death has been declared, there is no chance for recovery. The legal time of death is when the final diagnosis of brain death has been documented in the hospital chart.

We give advice, many donations; now can go again donations for good cause.

Tissue transplantation: Tissue donation is a precious gift. Ideally, the best replacement tissue following trauma, disease or surgery is the patients own tissue (autograft).

Banked tissues.

Eliminate the risks and expense of the additional incision necessary for acquiring an autograft

Prevent the creation of a permanent defect in the tissue recovery site.

Provide the surgeon with a varity and quantity of tissue that otherwise may bot be available, especially in children.

To provide safe, reliable and cost effective tissues for transplantation.

To offer training for the setting up of tissue bank.

To assist health authorities in developing guidelines and regulations for tissue banking.

To conduct research to enhance the properties of tissue transplantations.

To promote tissue donation.

A break through to boost liver transplantation: Currently, transplantation depends on preserving donor organs by putting them on ice, cooling them to slow their metabolism. But this often leads to organ becoming damaged. So the procedure, which will be a major boon for countries like India that already face an acute shortage of donor liver for transplantation. The innovation is a machine a device which keeps organ "alive and warm outside human body for 24 hours. A donated human liver connected to the device is raised to body temperature and oxygenated red blood cells are circulated through the capillaries. Once on a machine, a liver functions normally just as it would inside a human body, regaining its color and producing bile.

Mothers following the birth of thir babies donate *amniotic membranes*.

Persons undergoing primary joint replacement surgery, treatment for a femoral neck fracture, or trauma surgery donate musculoskeletal tissues.

Tissue is donated posthumously from decreased donors with the consent of the next of kin.

Safety of allograft: The donors blood is screened to rule out HIV/AIDS, hepatitis B& C, and syphilis. The tissues are processed to destroy microorganism and reduce antigen city preserved by freezing or freez drying and packaged in a sterile environment. The final products are sterilized by gamma radiation at ISOMED, the ISO 9002 certified radiation plant of the govt of India. They have a shelf-life of 3 years and can be stored at room temperature as ready to use packs.

Immune reaction: There are no problems of rejection as the transplantation antigen is destroyed during processing. Tissue typing is therefore, not necessary and antirejection drugs are not required in the recipient of the allograft.

Efficacy: Banked skin and amnion are excellent biological dressings and are used externally as temporary wound covers. Amnion requires no adhesives and peels off its own as healing progresses. Its use avoids the need for repeated, painful dressings, reduces the time of healing, and gives better long term results than routine dressings.

Banked amnion is used for—burns, ulcers, unresponsive bedsores and abscess. Leprosy lesions, skin graft donor sites and wounds, raw areas following dermabrasion and laser treatment, ocular surface and orbital defects, oral defects/ barrier membranes vaginoplasty.

Donated bone is among the most trans-planted tissues in the world, second only to blood. It is used to:

Reconstruct skeletal defects

Provide structural support during fracture healing particularly where there is non-union.

Reinforce bone that has been weakened as in patients with osteoarthritis and those under going revision joint replacement surgery.

Correct spinal deformities

Treat spinal defects resulting from the removal of tumors.

Replace cancerous bone enabling patients to stand and walk normally again sometimes preventing the amputation of a limb.

Chapter 13

Nurse with a Glance on Urinary System

Anatomy and Phsiology of Urinary System

The urinary system is composed of two kidneys, two tubes called ureters, one urinary bladder, and another tube called the urethra.

You probably know that the kidneys filter blood, so are a couple of blood vessels attached directly to each kidney. The full names of these vessels are the *renal artery and the renal vein.* Three of the four major metabolic wastes produced by the body are filtered from the blood by the kidneys. They are water, salts, and urea (the 4th, carbon dioxide, is excreted by the lungs. These are the same three wastes that sweat glands filter and excrete.

Each kidney (which can be thought of as BIG filters) is made up of thousands of tiny filtering sub-units called nephrons. The ureters are simply tubes that carry urine from the kidneys to the urinary bladder. The bladder temporarily stores urine. And the urethra is the tube through which urine leaves the body when you go for urination.

The urinary system consists of two kidneys, two ureters, the bladder and urethra. The kidneys are the primary functional structures in which urine is formed. The ureters are drainage tubes, which transmit the urine from the kidneys to the bladder where it is temporarily stored. The urethra is a duct that carries the urine to the exterior surface of the body.

Renal Functions

Overall function: Homeostasis the maintenance of a suitable environment for optimum cellular function

1. Regulation of fluid volume
2. Conservation of appropriate amounts of essential substances
3. Excretion of end products of metabolism, excesses, toxic substances and drugs
4. Regulation of the pH of body fluids by the elimination of non-volatile acids
5. Endocrine secretion of rennin, erythropoietin and active vitamin D

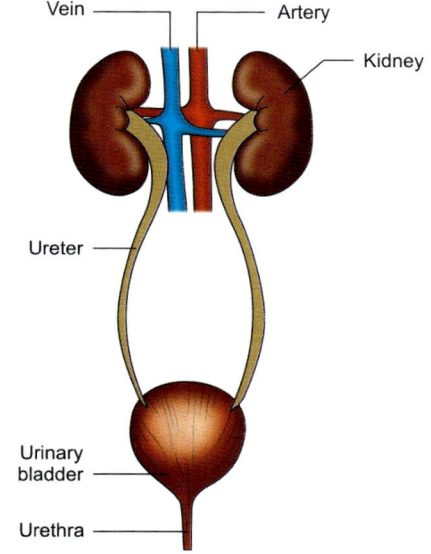

Fig. 13.1: Anatomy of urinary system

Presenting Symptoms/Clinical Manifestation

1. Change in the pattern of urinary elimination such as frequency, nocturia, difficulty initiating the stream of urine, inability to control urinary output, bed-wetting.
2. Changes in the volume in urinary output
3. Changes in color, odor
4. Pain and discomfort associated with voiding
5. Sensory changes related to the urge to void
6. Chills and fever
7. General symptoms like edema, headache, lethargy, fatigue, visual disturbances, loss of appetite and nausea.

Factors Influencing Urinary System Functions

1. Past experience and attitude
2. Diet and fluid intake
3. Lifestyle
4. Activity, mobility and dexterity
5. Level of awareness and orientation
6. Medications

Diagnostic Procedures

1. Urine examination
2. Blood chemistry determination

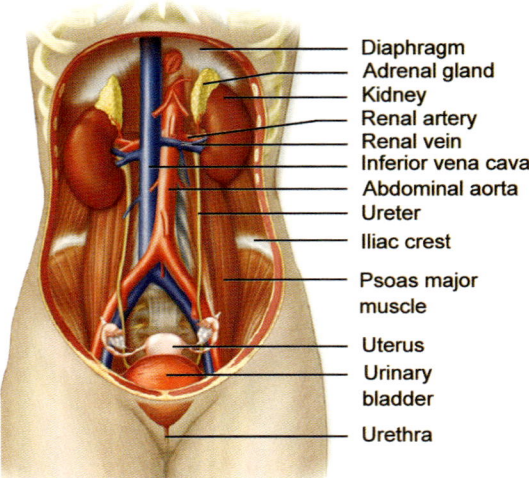

3. Hematological tests
4. Renal function test
5. Glomerular filtration rate
6. Renal scan
7. Intravenous (excretory) urogram
8. Ultrasound
9. Cystoscopy and retrograde pyelogram
10. Computerized axial tomography
11. Renal angiography
12. Nuclear magnetic resonance imaging
13. Percutaneous renal biopsy
14. Retrograde renal brush biopsy
15. Uridynamic investigations

Identification of patient's problems—change in pattern of urinary elimination: Urinary tract infection, bladder calculi, emotional stress, neurological disorders, disorders of urinary formation.

Alteration in pattern of urinary elimination incontinence: Urethral sphincter incompetence, detrusor muscle instability, impaired neurological control of maturation, pelvic floor disorders, congenital anomalies of urinary system, loss of cerebral awareness, urinary tract infection.

Alteration in pattern of urinary elimination-retention: Obstructive disease of the bladder or urethra, surgical intervention, neurological disease, embarrassment or fear.

Impaired renal function: Renal dysfunction may be due to a primary disease within the kidneys or may be secondary to a disorder elsewhere in the body. The body is dependent on the kidneys for the elimination of metabolic wastes and maintenance of homeostasis. When kidney function is impaired, dysfunction of external systems ultimately develops. Similarly, primary dysfunction in other systems may readily affect renal function.

Renal failure: When the kidneys are unable to excrete metabolic wastes and perform their

Labels for figure:
Diaphragm
Adrenal gland
Kidney
Renal artery
Renal vein
Inferior vena cava
Abdominal aorta
Ureter
Iliac crest
Psoas major muscle
Uterus
Urinary bladder
Urethra

Fig. 13.2: Organs of abdominal cavity

Table 13.1: Actual and potential problems of the patient with acute renal failure

Problem	Contributing factors	Goals
Alteration in fluid volume excess	Inability of the kidneys to excrete water	To achieve fluid balance
Alteration in nutritional status and needs; change related to body requirements and retention of metabolic waste	Inability of the kidneys to excrete catabolic nitrogenous waste and excess electrolytes	To achieve and maintain adequate nutrition and electrolyte balance
Protein impairment of oral mucosa and skin integrity	Edema and increased excretion of water through the skin	To maintain the integrity of the skin and oral mucosa
Potential for infection	Effect or uremia on the constituents of the blood	To prevent infection and bleeding
Anxiety	Sudden onset of illness	To decrease anxiety
Potential for injury	Alteration level of awareness	To prevent injury
Alteration in fluid volume deficit	Fluid loss	To maintain fluid and electrolyte balance
Lack of knowledge about plans for discharge and follow upcare	Inadequate knowledge	To develop plans for home management and follow upcare

role in fluid, electrolyte and acid–base balance, renal failure exists.

Acute renal failure: Acute renal failure is a sudden, severe interruption of kidney function that in most instances is a complication of another disorder and is reversible.

Chronic renal failure: Chronic renal failure is due to progressive disease of both kidneys. Irreversible damage to nephrons occurs which eventually leads to the retention of many waste and toxic products of metabolism, fluid and electrolyte imbalances, metabolic acidosis, anemia, hypertension and decalcification of bone tissue.

Causes

1. Glomerulonephritis
2. Polycytic kidney disease
3. Nephrosclerosis
4. Drug and anal analgesic abuse

Physiological disturbances caused by chronic renal failure

1. Fluid and electrolyte disturbances
2. Cardiovascular and pulmonary disturbances
3. Neurological disturbances
4. Gastrointestinal disturbances
5. Hematological disturbances
6. Musculoskeletal disturbances

Chapter 14

Example of Routine Activities

Routine activities carried out in AKD unit according to time/shift (each hospital has their unique plan and policy they follow, this activities in hospital where I worked. It is important to the novice student for whom it is a different world for the first time when she enters the department with cross fingers and lack of confidence without any experience).

6.00 am Batch One—Shift One

1. Keep the files according to clients number
2. Take note of injection heparin
3. Keep the boxes (dialyzer = tubing) according to number
4. Check files for number of dialysis, number of dialyzer, number of tubing
5. Check for any injection, e.g. iron and hemoglobin and write down the prescription (any replacement—prescription for client
6. Check for any blood test and write down the prescription and keep ready the blood tubes with label and pathology form
7. Keep in heparin ready for all client
8. Once machines are ready call the client according to the number
9. Check the weight, take sitting BP and lying down BP and make a record in the file, in clients card and in the book (same procedure for all 10 clients)
10. If any catheter client is there we do the clients cleansing and dressing
11. Any blood collection has to be done it is mentioned on the board and take the blood samples and sent it to the pathology department. It is recorded in clients file and the register where too documentation is done.
12. Any client has any health problem, e.g. high BP, vomiting, giddiness, it is informed to sister in charge and needful action is taken. This client observed and checked every 2 hourly BP.
13. After confirming clients are offered tea or coffee from the canteen and served to client, if client needs assistance to have coffee and biscuits he is helped.
14. Inventory is checked and all things need for the day is kept ready.
15. If any admitted client sister in charge is informed
16. Then the recording/reading from machine are charted in the file and department register (e.g. BP, venous pressure, VF rate, blood flow)
17. Then BP is checked one hourly, if client has any complaint like headache, sweating the BP, and RBS is checked and as per need 25% dextrose 100 ml is given and recorded in file, registers of department to be replaced.
18. With the receipt register book is maintained
19. Next dialysis appointments noted

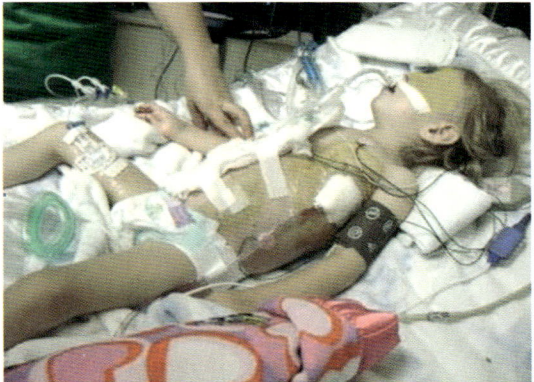
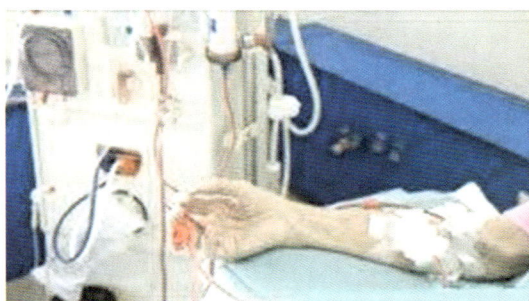
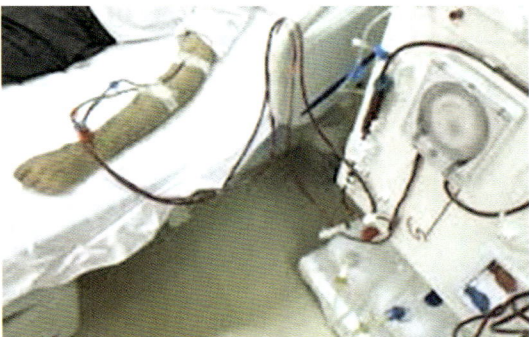
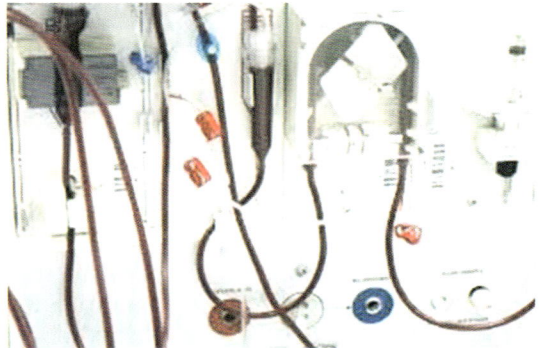
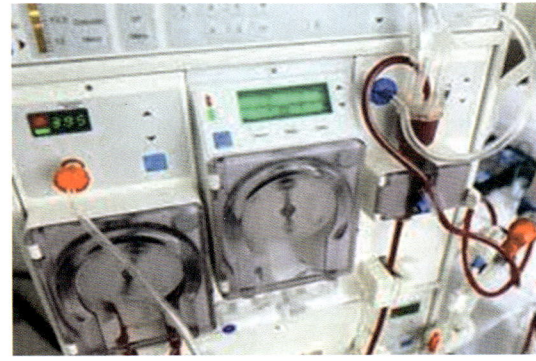
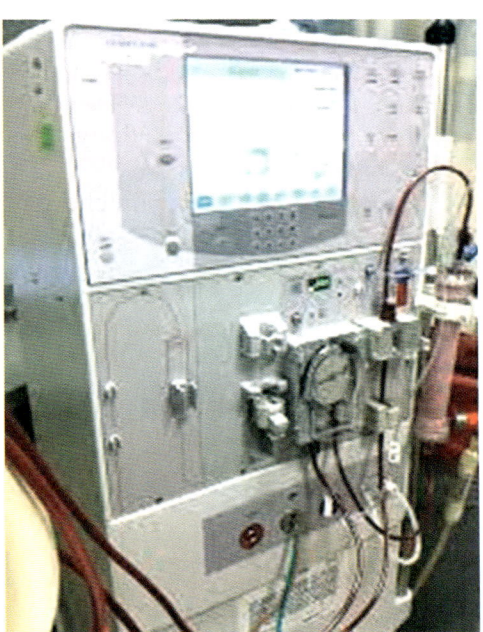
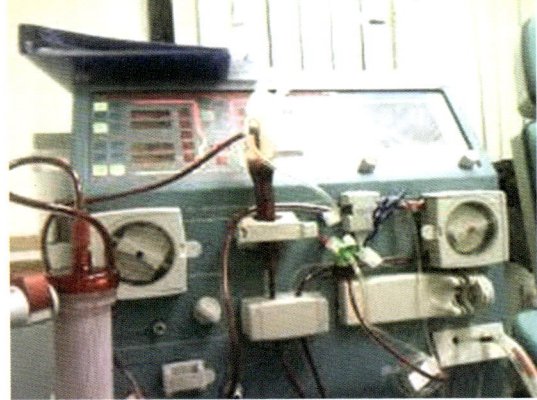

Fig. 14.1: Dialysis unit set (routine activities)

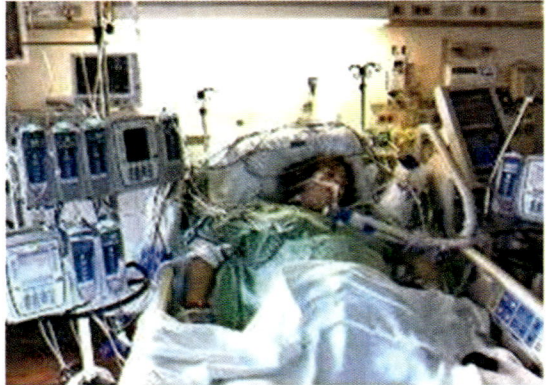
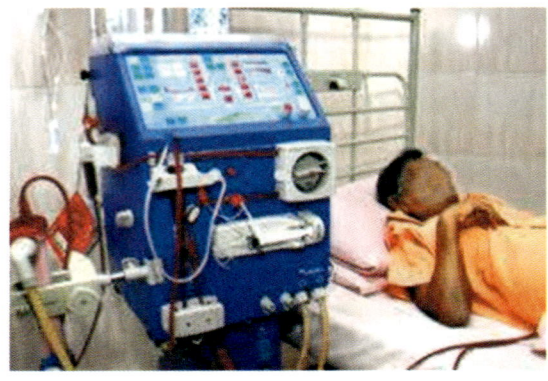
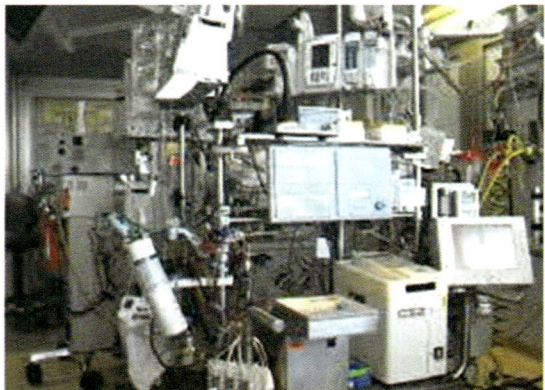
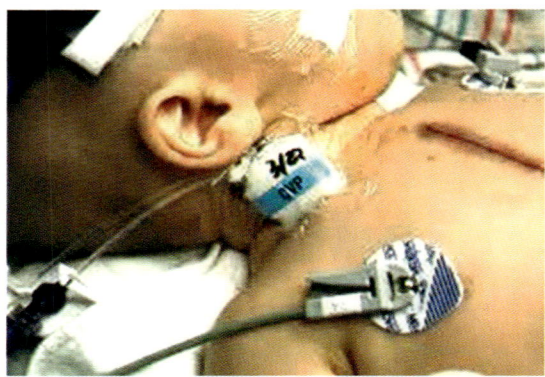
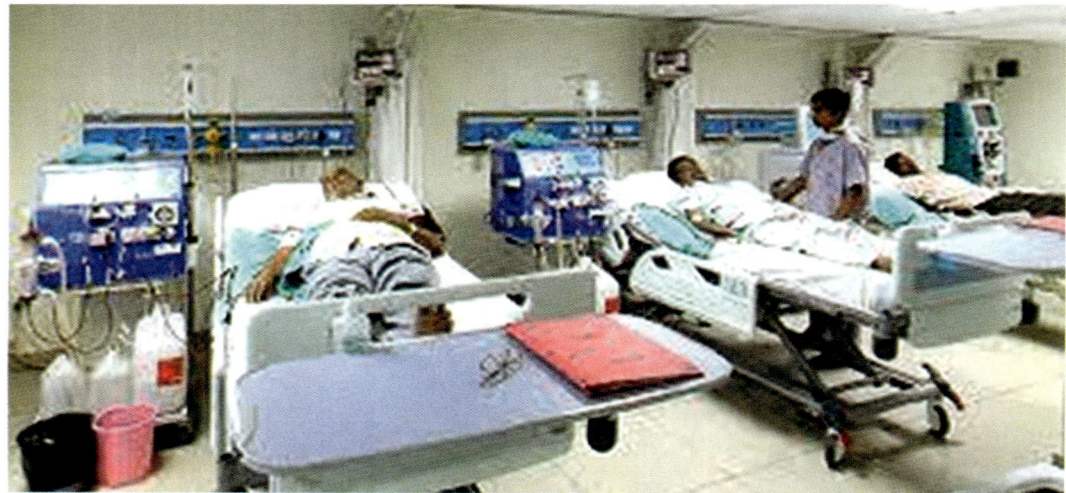

Fig. 14.2: Department of dialysis and client under HD procedure

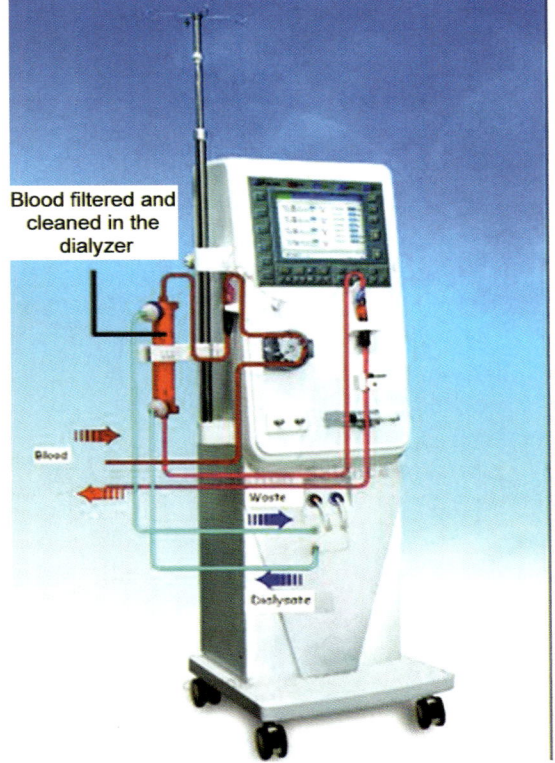

Blood filtered and cleaned in the dialyzer

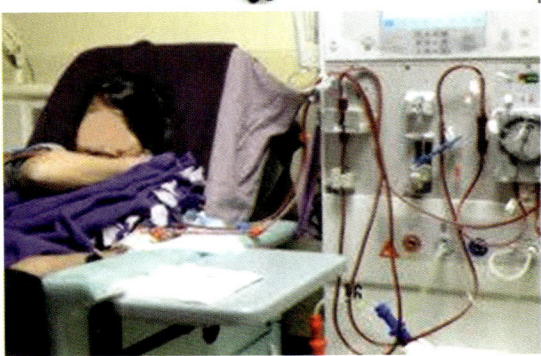

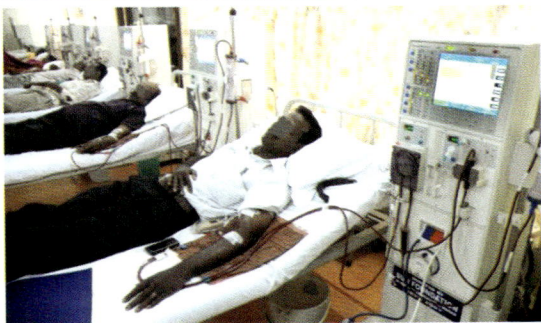

Fig. 14.3: Dialysis machine and client undergoing HD procedure

20. Around 9.00 am a breakfast is ordered to clients who wants to have.

21. Files are checked for next batch, e.g. injection heparin and injection iron, and prescriptions are written down. To give handover the files and kept in order of the clients timings.

22. When one hour remains for first batch, injection iron and is administered, when last 20 minutes are left injection erythropoietin is given.

23. All dialyzer, tubing boxes, injection heparin, 100 ml N/S with saline set is kept ready.

24. All the reports attached to the file for physicians ward round.

25. Regular intervals vitals are checked and entered into nurses notes

26. Once dialysis is completed and need taken out once again BP, weight, checked and in file, client's card, register note is done. Client is given explanation for his next appointment timings.

1st Batch—at 11.00 am

1. Call the client according to number and check BP, weight in both sitting and lying position. It is recorded in clients card and in register and department file.

2. In any health problem noted sister in charge is informed, and clients vitals are checked half hourly.

3. Appointment and name is entered in register and medication that client has brought is entered into the file.

4. Same as above at 11.00 am articles like dialyzer, tubing boxes, 100 ml N/S with saline sets are kept ready for the batch.

5. Client is served tea, biscuits, and same as above observations and noted.

2nd Batch

1. Handover from 1st shift staff done. All the files checked as morning shift.

2. Inventory is checked

3. File is checked for injection and prescriptions. Client is handover, replacement is kept ready
4. All the files are cheeked for appointment and injection entry is done
5. Nurses notes are completed
6. At 3.00 pm to 3.30 pm is time for termination. Once again vitals are checked and same as above procedure is followed
7. Checked BP, weight, and noted in file, register and clients card
8. Now cots are kept ready for 3.30 pm batch, procedure repeated the same sequences
9. When the 3rd batch is going on
10. Keep the unit ready for 7.30 batch
11. All files are checked and for next days batch unit is kept ready-for investigations, right blood test, HIV, HBsAg and HCV, vaccine to be done for the next day and prescription sheet, flowchart and nursing sheet and all necessary things are checked and changed.
12. All the names of the next day's client's names are written on the board.
13. When doctor comes for round if any changes of medication explain to client and record in information register.
14. Vitals are checked hourly, if any injection inferon and injection erythropoietin administered last 15 minutes.
15. Before termination once again vitals are checked and once needle is out BP, weight checked and recorded. Client is explained for next appointment.
16. For 7.30 pm batch unit is kept ready and same procedure carried out (Monday and Saturday clients will be there)

3rd Batch

1. Handover taken as 2nd shift
2. Inventory checked
3. Clients appointments are checked
4. All clients BP is checked and recorded
5. For morning shift all equipment like dialyzer tubing, all boxes, N/S 100 ml, IV set, fistula needles, heparin syringes, fistula trays on each bedside.
6. See that registered is completed and all documentations are done.
7. Night ward boy is asked to do proper cleaning and department is kept neat and tidy.
8. All the machines are checked, AC, fans and light are put off
9. Night ward boy is instructed to make Dialysis cans ready for use in the morning
10. Dressing trolley is checked and all articles needed for next day kept ready
11. Fistula and catheter tray is kept ready according to dates.
12. At 5.30 am N/S with sets are collected.

Activities

1. Machines servicing done regularly on every 4th month (we have three different company machines such as nipro-hamoclam solution used for it, fresenius machine where cirtostend solution used, B-Brown machine citric acid solution is used).
2. Each morning machines are checked and then primed before putting client on dialysis.
3. Each night machines are formalized from time.
4. HIV, HCV, HbsAg status of all clients checked every.
5. Clients and educated and informed in details and their consent obtained before dialysis.
6. Fistula puncture by needles under aseptic care by nurses/technicians.
7. Before and after procedure clients weight checked on digital machine.
8. Tourniquet are tied at puncture site after putting antiseptic powder.
9. All AKD staffs follow universal safety guidelines.
10. Any separate COTS dedicated for Hepatitis "B" and "C" and their dialyzers are cleaned in separate wash basin.

11. All emergency drugs and trolleys are checked and updated daily. Central oxygen and central suction are also checked daily.
12. Regular swabs and Reverse Osmosis (RO) and dialysate water are sent for colony forming units (CFU) and endotoxin (EU).

Documentation

- Document condition and appearance of dialysis catheter site at least every shift
- Document heparin flushes on the medication order sheet
- Dialysis catheters, when de-clotted by the dialysis nurse using TPA, document verification of occlusion, volume of TAP instilled, number of attempts required, result of instillation, and clients response in the medical record. Document dosage of TPA on medication order sheet
- Document client/family education on the teaching record
- Maintained dialysis unit client ID card record details such as (date, client name, address, phone number, consulting nephrologists, diagnosis, Australian antigen, blood grouping, HIV anti-body, date of HD, pre-dialysis weight—BP, post-dialysis weight—BP, unique small diary record entered).

Management of Clinet Care

1. Physical examination observing, recording and reporting of vitals to concerned doctor
2. ABCs-check the vital signs and recorded access sites
3. Inspection of AV fistula site (palpated for thrills, listen for bruits)
4. Shave and clean the area before inserting needles
5. Do not use affected extremity for BP or venipuncture to prevent bruising, bleeding and risk for infection
6. Keep site and extremity warm, advise client to wash it daily with antibacterial soap and water.
7. Watch for any complication during dialysis and inform consultant
8. Post-dialysis remove the fistula needles and give pressure on needle site with gauze pieces, apply antibiotic powder/ointment and tie with tourniquet.
9. Explain client to remove the tourniquet after 4–6 hours and in between watch for oozing
10. Educated client and relatives' how to untie the tourniquet at home
11. Instructed client to take daily weight and record accurate intake, output, check for any scales or blood clotting, fever, redness, swelling, pain on fistula site
12. Avoid soap for bathing to prevent drying skin, use oil in bath water
13. Doctor should be seen immediately if the access site bleeds or catheter becomes dislodged
14. Avoid wearing constructive clothing or ornaments, watch over the access site
15. Take regular medications as per advised by the doctor.

Chapter 15

Records and Equipment of Unit

Hospital Printed Records (Materials) Maintained by Nursing Staff

1. AKD registration book (AKD payment book—Daily dialysis record book)
2. Daily consumed stock record book pharmacy and store
3. Daily inventory book with three monthly expiry book
4. Replacement book
5. Dialysis department investigation report, blood test register
6. Dialysis department hemodialysis chart—consultant Nephrologists file
7. Staff assignment register
8. Information register (communication register)
9. Washing and on call register
10. Repairing information register
11. Pharmacy expiry register
12. AMC/serving machines register
13. Waiting list register
14. Store register
15. CSSD register
16. Fumigation register
17. Others as each hospital policy

Hospital Printed Records Materials Attached to the Client's Case File

1. Consent form
2. Flow sheet of blood
3. Investigation form number 03
4. Dialysis flow chart form number 02
5. Treatment sheet
6. Nurses notes records

Equipment of AKD

1. Hemodialysis machine
2. Crash Cart
3. BP apparatus, stethoscope
4. Central supply suction
5. Monitor
6. Laryngoscope with blades
7. Glucometer
8. Suction machines
9. Continuous renal replacement therapy (CRRT) machine
10. Reverse osmosis filter and charcoal
11. Ventilator

Other Articles

1. Masks
2. Sterile gloves
3. Syringes, 20 cc (2)
4. Sterile normal saline
5. Dressing set/gauze
6. Povidone solution
7. Towel
8. Sterile bowl
9. Heparin 25,000 iu
10. Nonsterile glove
11. Xylocaine for local anesthesia

12. Fistulae needle
13. Dialysis machine, tubing
14. Dialyser
15. Dialysate solution
16. Tourniquet

Requirements of Unit

1. Dialysis machines with filter
2. RO plant
3. Dialyser and tubing
4. Fistula needles/double luman catheters
5. Monitoring devices, e.g. NIBP, glucometer, BP instrument
6. Trained dialysis technicians and nursing staff
7. Reuse room
8. Separate machines reuse room and staff for positive patients
9. Materials like bicarbonate and acid cans, NS, heparin, etc.

PATIENT

Vascular Access with Good Blood Flow

1. Consent form for dialysis and related procedure
2. Forms to record medical history including investigations and medications
3. Format to record pre/intra and post dialytic events
4. Patients feedback form
5. Shiftwise check list
6. Form for new patient
7. Patient's reference form
8. Records

The equipment used in the department include:
- Hemodialysis machines
- RO system
- Monitoring devices like—NIBP, glucometer, BP instument, weighing machine, pulse oxemeter.

Procedure: For equipment breakdown

All malfunctioning equipment will be removed from use and send for repair.

Hemodialysis machine/RO system

1. Defective/malfunction tagging must be done.
2. Inform biomedical department on extension: 1353/54
3. Patients with prior appointments, who are already in, should be informed about the same. They should be told immediately about next possible alternative and the time taken for arrangement of the alternative.
4. Next day's appointments should be rescheduled and sick, admitted patient, female patient and elderly patients should be given priority.

Weight Machine/BP Apparatus/ECG Machine/Defibrillator/Nebulisation Machine/Pulse Oximeter

1. Defective/malfunction tagging must be done. Inform medical and administrative HOD immediately.
2. Inform biomedical department on extension.
3. Obtain alternate machine from other unit on temporary basis or through biomedical department.

Operation Theater Techniques

Chapter 16

Three Phases of Surgery

Operation Theater

The success of every surgery depends on the type of nursing care given to the client before, during and after period of surgery.

The preparation of clients for surgery depends on the type of surgery, age of client, general health of client and organ involved.

Surgery is the oldest and most widely used method and treatment, today surgical techniques have improved, full collaboration between nurses, doctors and other health care professionals is vital if the patent has to be restored back.

The word surgery was synonymous with knife and cutting, surgeon who removes organ or parts of organ, limbs from the body, but with the passage of time many surgical procedure have become more refined with progress there have come many changes, future generations of surgeons may marvel at the audacity and removing that of all progress in medicines. Many abnormalities found throughout the body. The surgeon informing the patient of the diagnosis, prognosis and operative procedure. Continued research and development of new techniques, equipment and drug is helping to enhance the prognosis.

THEATER TECHNIQUE

Theater Dress

1. All persons entering the actual theater must change into theater clothing and into-static shoes should be worn
2. Trousers suits, tie shirt and pant it is practical, comfortable and flattering
3. Cotton has been the material of choice for theater clothes as it allows both circulation of air over the body and evaporation from the skin
4. Use of anti-static foot wear
5. Use of overshoes is to be discouraged
6. Use of disposable masks is effective for up to two and half hours
7. If use of cotton masks then it should be fiber free, light weight and comfortable
8. Mask should be changed at the end of a long operation and discarded on leaving theater.

Theater Head Wear

1. All staff working within the actual theater must ensure that their hair is completely covered
2. Disposable hats are popular because they are light weight and comfortable to wear and they do not interfere with hearing
3. Beards should be covered by wearing a second mask

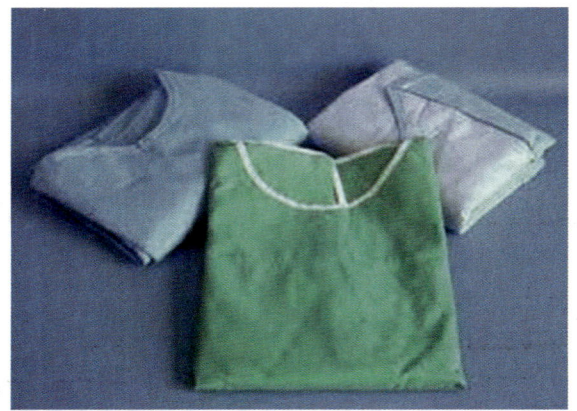

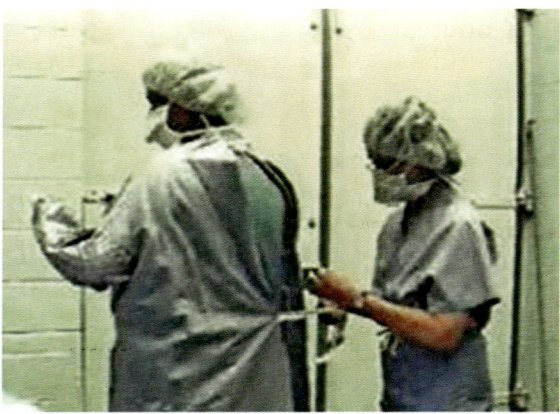

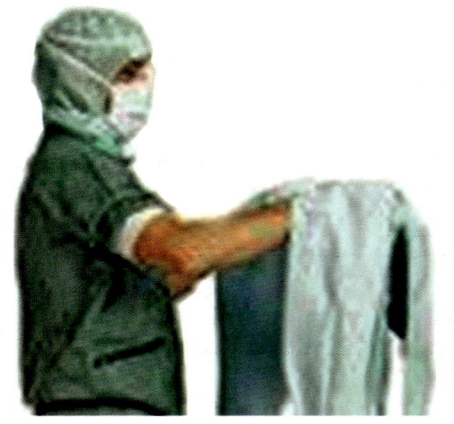

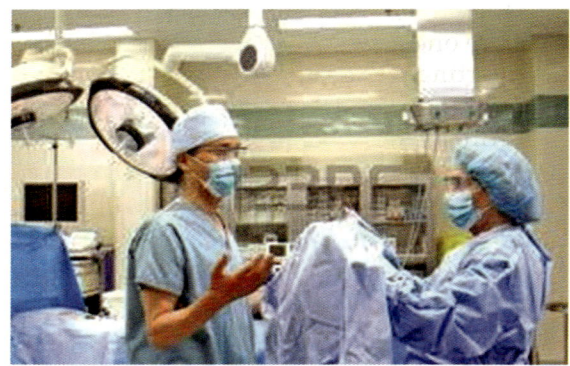

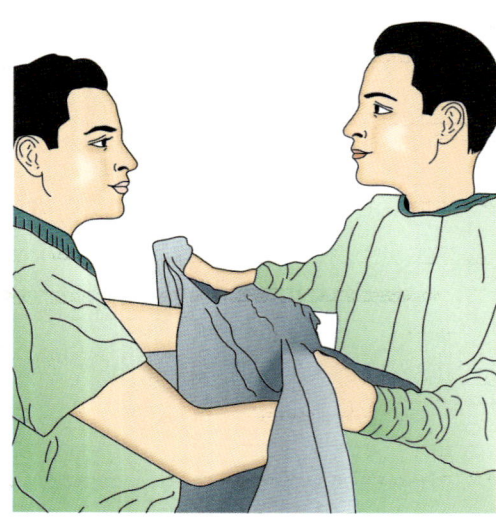

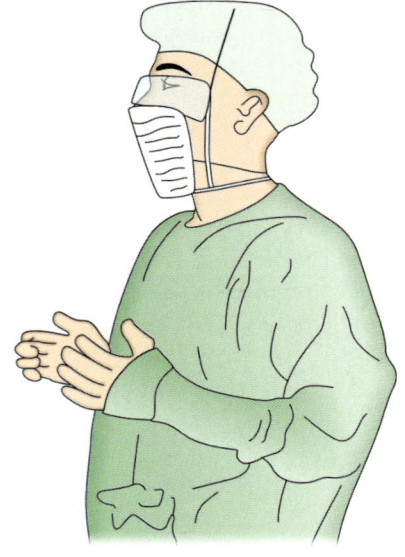

Fig. 16.1: Technique of sterile gowning

4. If nondisposable head wear is worn if should be lightweight to allow air to circulate freely for continued comfort.

Hand Washing and Gowning

1. The first hand wash of the day should last for 5 minutes or as long as it takes to ensure that hands are both socially clean and disinfected.
2. Nails should be short and nail polish should not be worn.
3. Weak chemical agents can safely be used for hand washing provided there is no skin cut or abrasion.
   a. Pick up one towel so that it remains folded in half length wise
   b. Use one end of the towel to dry the hand starting with the fingers
   c. Use the other end of the towel to dry the arm, using a slower circular notion never return to an area which has been dried
   d. Repeat the procedure for the other hand
   e. Discard the towel
   f. Pick up the gown firmly. It should be packed inside out to avoid the risk of toweling the outside with the ungloved hand
   g. Find the top of the gown (it is useful to have an indicator on gowns. It can be colored tab or a mark denoting the top)
   h. Hold the gown securely as it unfolds
   i. Bring the armholes into view and insert the arms
   j. Work both arms into the gown at the same time (if the closed method of gloving is being used, push the hands to the inner edge of the cuff only. For the open method of gloving, push the hands through the cuffs).
   k. The circular will be tie the back tapes of the gown

Gloving

A. Closed Method

The circular will open the outer pack of the sterilized gloves

1. With the thumb and fore finger collect the glove pack from inside the gown
2. Put the pack on the sterile towel and open flat
3. Thorough the gown, grasp the right glove with the left hand. Turn to right hand so that the palm is upward
4. Place the palm of the glove to the palm of the hands, with the thumb of the glove over the thumb of the hand
5. Grasp the palm side of the glove cuff with thumb and fore finger, through the gown
6. With the left hand, still inside the cuff, grasp the top cuff of the glove and pull it over the fingers.
7. Push the fingers into the glove, grasp the sleeve and glove and pull on
8. Repeat the procedure for the left hand
9. Gloves can now be adjusted

B. Open Method

When the gown is put on the hands are pull through the cuffs

1. The glove packed is collected from the circular and placed flat on the sterile towel
2. The packet of powder is removed from the glove pack and the hands are powdered
3. Pick up the left glove with the right hand by the inside turned down cuff
4. Carefully push the fingers of the left hand into the glove until it reaches the cuff
5. Pick up the right glove by putting the gloved hand under the cuff
6. Carefully push the fingers of the right hand into the glove and pull the glove cuff of the gown
7. Now pull the cuff on the left glove completely over the gown cuff of the left hand
8. Adjust the gloves

C. Plunge Method

This method can only be used when one person is already gloved and gowned

1. Pick up the glove with a gloved hand

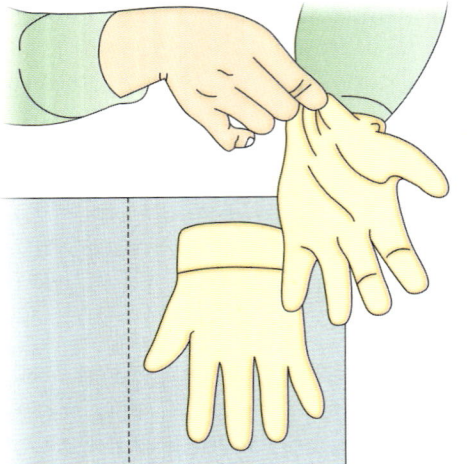

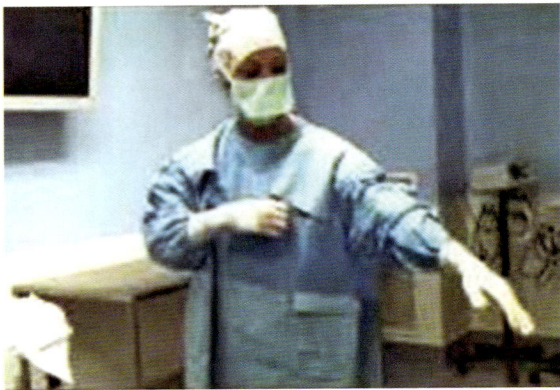

Fig. 16.2: Surgical gloving

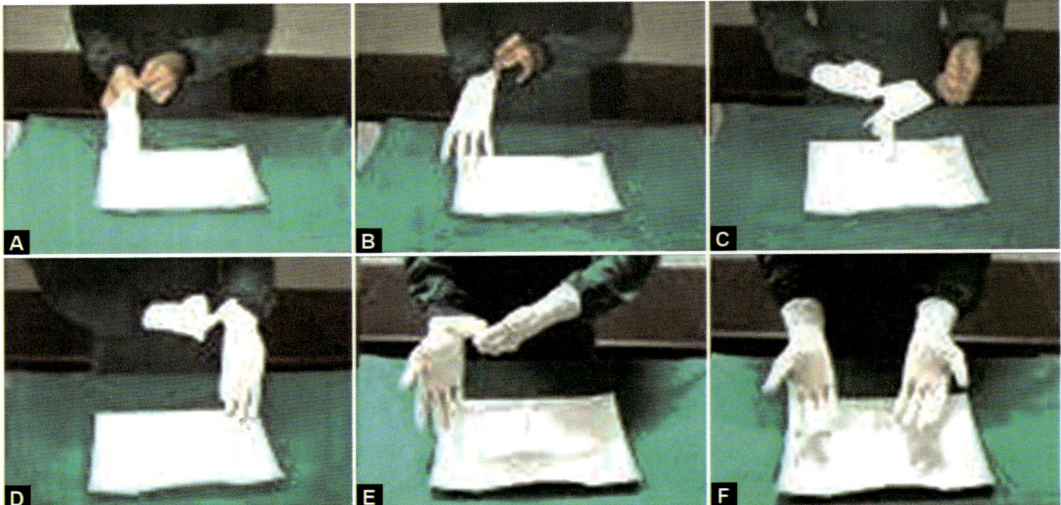

Fig. 16.3: Surgical gloving procedure

2. Insert the finger of both hands under the cuff of the glove and hold it open

3. Position the glove under the opened hand of the other person, glove thumb facing their thumb

4. The other person now plunges his hand into the glove while the gloved person puts it completely over the gown cuff.

Nurse's Role

1. Reached to see that there is no pressure point and no constriction which might damage nerves or blood vessels when the patient has been placed in the position for the procedure

2. All tubing (BP cuff, IV solution of urinary drainage) should be checked to be certain it is not obstructed by the patients position

3. If the electrosurgical unit is to be used place the conductive plate under the patient with a broad area of skin contact.

Surgical Team

1. Receptionist

2. Surgeon
3. Housekeeping anesthetist
4. Scrub nurse
5. Technician
6. Assistant surgeon
7. Assistant anesthetist
8. Store keeper
9. Circulatory nurse
10. Technician

Let us understand the infrastructure in figure form the operation theater that will help in one glance the operation theater set up.

Surgery is a unique experience of a planned physical alteration encompassing three phases of surgery as follows:
1. Preoperative phase
2. Intraoperative phase
3. Postoperative phase

Preoperative Client's Preparation

Preoperative phase begins with when the decision to have a surgery is made; it ends when the client is transferred to the operating table.

Definition: Preoperative care of the client begins as soon as the surgeon makes a diagnosis and decides that an operation is necessary for the client.

Purposes

1. To prevent infection
2. To remove the fear from clients mind
3. To promote psychological well-being
4. To prevent complications

Purposes of Surgical Procedures

1. *Diagnostic*—confirms or establishes a diagnosis
2. *Palliative*—relieves or reduces pain or symptoms of a disease, it does not cure
3. *Ablative*—removed a diseased body part.
4. *Constructive*—restores function or appearance that has been lost or reduced
5. *Transplant*—replaces malfunctioning structures.

Preoperative Checklist and Nurse's Role

1. *Identification* data—name, age, sex, IP No. ward, bed no. diagnosis, surgery proposed, date of surgery.
2. *Collection of nursing history*—medical history, previous surgeries, clients and family members perceptions and understanding of surgery, medication, history of allergies, habits like smoking and alcohol, family support, occupation, etc.
3. *Review of clients* and family members emotional health—anxiety, their doubts, clarification
4. *Physical examination of client*—general appearance, physical measures, height, weight, vital signs, head to toe examination, neurological examination, etc.
5. Identification and *analysis of risk factors*—age, nutrition, fluid and electrolyte balance.
6. *Diagnostic* screening.

Day Prior to Surgery

1. Weight, height, known allergy, medication consumed (specific)
2. Consent for surgery is obtained in specified format (the nature and the reason for the surgery)
3. Teaching about preoperative exercise given
4. Explain about anesthesia and surgery given
5. Surgical preparation of the skin
6. Enema/bowel wash given
7. Recoding done about any cough/alteration in vital signs/loose teeth/skin infection/menstruation/any others
8. X-rays, scan, ECG, lab reports, etc. collected and attached to clients record (explain the need for preoperative tests)
9. Instruction given about fasting
10. Types of cross-match for blood done
11. Consent for receiving blood transfusion obtained.
12. Notify surgeon for any abnormal lab report.

OT infrastructure figures will bring in front of the eyes the inside scenario of the operation theater

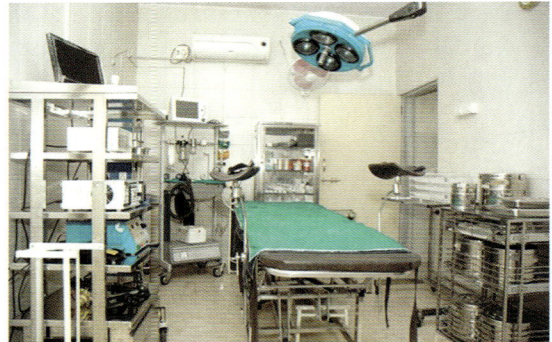
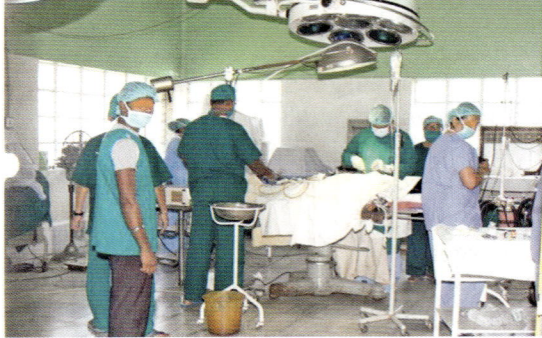
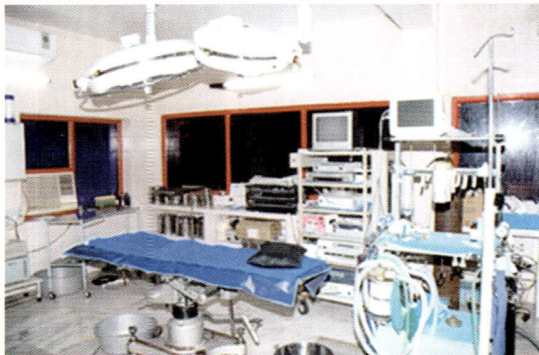
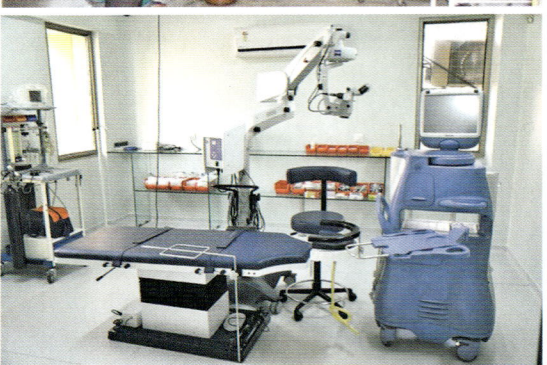
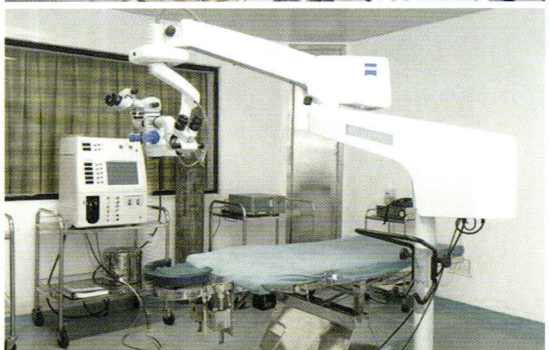
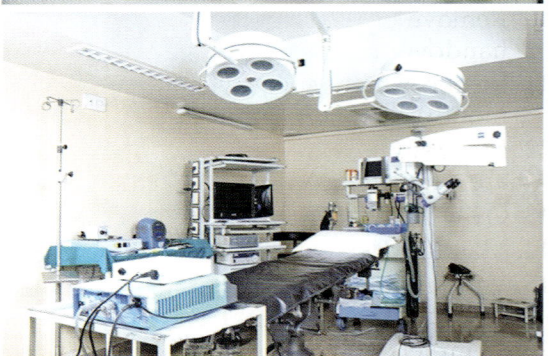
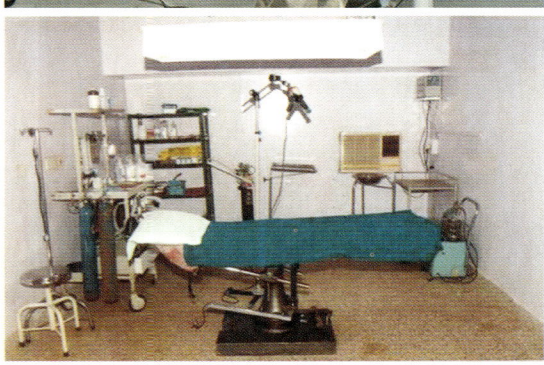
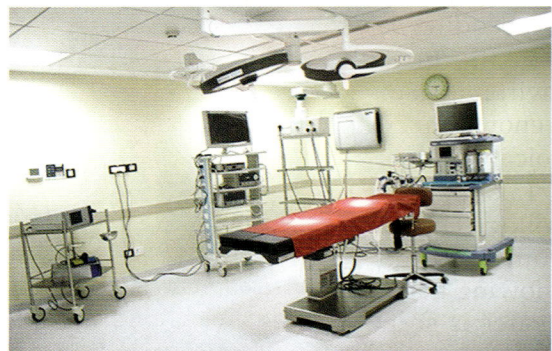

Fig. 16.4: Operation unit setting

13. Psychological preparation (types of surgery, consequences of surgery, expected duration of hospitalization, cost of surgery)

Preoperative Client's Preparation

1. Eradication fear of operation from client (explain what happens during anesthesia, explain how to get rid of pain after surgery, tell when he can take meals)
2. Meet the spiritual needs of the client
3. Check the physicians order for the diagnosis and order of operation
4. Check informed consent
5. Fitness for operation should be ensured
6. Arrange for reserved blood if required
7. Provide psychological reassurance
8. Prepare skin on particular site of operation which is very important to reduce number of micro-organism and reduce the possibility of wound infection
9. Shave the required operative area, clean with antiseptic solution
10. Remove jewelry, cosmetics, dentures, and handover to the relative
11. Re-check the requirement of NBM (nil by month) status to client
12. Make sure that the preoperative changes are deposited
13. OT clothes should be given to client
14. Maintain personal hygiene of the client
15. Venous access, Foley's catheter insertion should be done as per doctor's advice
16. Complete the preoperative checklist
17. Sending the client to operating room

In the hospital, entering the strange environment of the hospital for ones surgery is enough to create anxiety in even the most stoic individuals.

Take patient to the operating room on a trolley. The operating room looks sinister from a horizontal position to everyone. Knowing that the first sight of the operating theater is scary to most people, and prior knowledge of what to expect may help reduce your anxiety. The operating room is cold and sterile. People appear with uniforms, caps and masks, strong lights are focused on you from different directions. You will be linked up to some of these machines, which may make different beeps and sounds. Doctors mat pick and pork your body and administer various drugs. However, instead of getting scared, you should feel reassured by the sterile atmosphere and all the machines since all this is geared towards one goal; your safety.

Know the various tubes in your body and the equipment around you: an intravenous line allows drugs and fluids to be administered to you. Heart monitor are constantly monitored, urinary catheter, Endotracheal tube, arterial line helps monitor blood pressure and measure the oxygenation of blood. Chest drainage tubes help drain blood from, oxygen mask, etc.

Overall Design

1. Entry at one side and exit at other to avoid across traffic and risk of infection.
2. Staff should have access to changing area from outside and patients can be admitted through a reception area for checking.
3. Lounges, stock room, linen rooms and other ancillary rooms should be located on the outside of the theater complex.
4. They should be separated from the actual theaters by a dividing corridor.
5. There should be direct entry to the theater from the anesthetic room.
6. A hatch from the theatre should allow for the disposal of used equipment collection
7. An area for preparation of equipment for surgery should be directly attached to the theater and the sinus for hand washing should be adjacent.

Day of Surgery

1. Confirm NBM status
2. Bowel preparation—enema/bowel wash given (if indicated)
3. Bath given

OT infrastructure figures will bring in front of the eyes the inside scenario of the operation theater

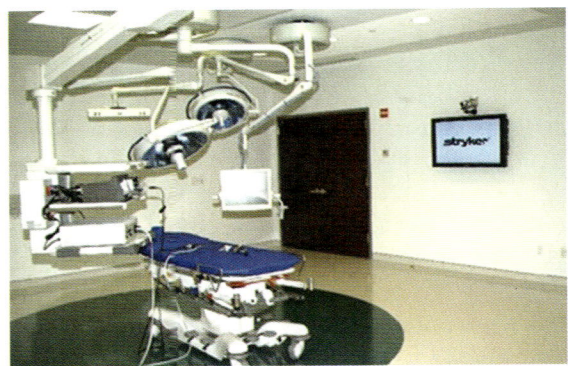
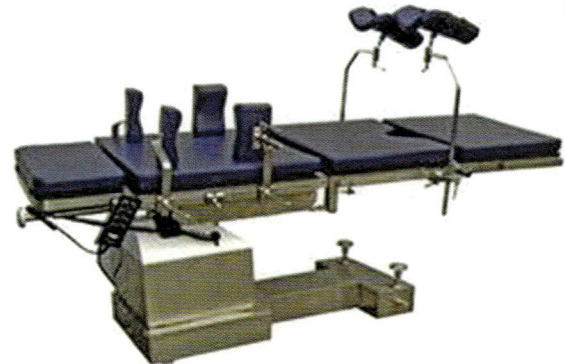
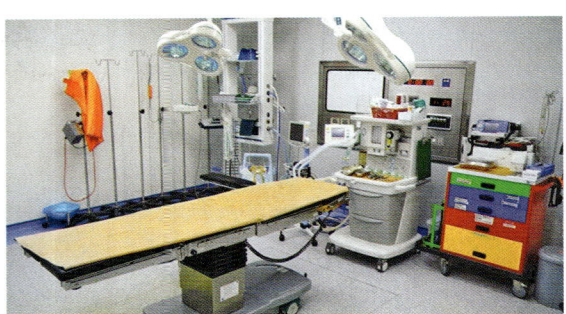
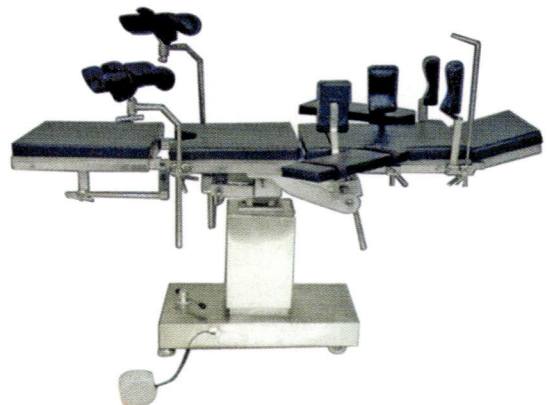

Fig. 16.5: OT tables

4. Final skin preparation done
5. Ryle's tube, catheterization, IV line, passed (if indicated)
6. Intraverous line is placed
7. Vital signs checked and recorded
8. Bladder emptied (catheterization if indicated)
9. Pre-medication given if ordered
10. Time recorded when client left the ward
11. Signature, date and time noted
12. Before sending to OT recheck the check list and sign by sister in charge and staff on duty
13. Transfer client to OT as per client's condition on either stretcher or wheel chair.

14. Give handover of the client to OT staff and take the sign on check list such as check clients all repots, medications, X-ray, ECG, CT scan and any other investigation ordered and sign.

Intraoperative care begins when the client is transferred to the operating table and end when the client is admitted to the post-anesthesia care unit.

1. When a client arrives in the operating room three groups of personnel are involved in the care—the anesthetic team, the surgical team, the operating room nurses
2. Intraoperative nurses are responsible for the safety and well-being of the client, the

co-ordination of the operating room personnel and activities of the circulating nurse and the scrub nurse.

3. The circulating nurse assures cleanliness, proper temperature. Humidity and lighting, the safe functioning of the equipment and the availability of the supplies and materials. And monitoring safety of the client throughout the surgical procedure.

4. Scrubbing for surgery, setting up the sterile tables, preparing sutures, ligatures and special equipment and assisting surgeons during procedure.

5. Check vitals such as take temperature, pulse, respiration, blood pressure, weight and record it in clients check list.

6. As per surgery time and type OT staff should prepare the anesthesia trolley, equipment, and instrument.

7. Before surgery carbonization of table should be done

8. Cover the clients hair, shift the client on the table, attach the monitors, start oxygen

9. Remove the clients clothes and cover clients with bedsheet

10. Prepare the skin and apply the Cutasept solution on the operation site (in orthopedic surgeries scrub with bets scrub and Savlon solution).

11. Set instrument as per required

12. Keep a check on Mobs, and needles, gauze, sutures counting properly used

13. Suture cutting should be done

14. Quaterise when needed

15. Be alert during operation

16. Record all the medications given, BT, removing of any fluid, done

17. After surgery is over dress the client, give comfortable position, and shift the client to recovery room.

18. Once vitals are stable and client becomes conscious, hand over client to the ward staff.

Postoperative care/General Postoperative Phase begin with the Admission of the Client to the Post-anesthesia Area and Ends when Healing is Complete

1. Preparation of post-anesthetic bed and reception of the client

2. Discuss pain management

3. Explain usual activity restrictions and precautions related to getting up for the first time postoperatively.

4. Describe usual dietary alterations

5. Discuss postoperative dressings and drains

6. Adequate number of people to transfer the client without disturbing the functioning of the devices attached with the client such as intravenous infusion set, self retaining suction set, blood transfusion set, nasogastric tube, oxygen urinary catheters, cardiac monitoring, water seal drainage system, plaster casts, traction sets.

7. Ask the theater staff who has accompanied with the client about any complications that has occurred in the operation room during surgery.

8. Before anesthetic return to operation theater the nurse checks the vitals sings, blood pressure, pulse rate, respiration, color of the skin and nails for any cyanosis, etc. compare it with the baseline data recorded before sending to operation theater.

9. Check the operation site for bleeding, discharge, etc. if drainage tubes are fitted

10. Keep the client well covered to prevent draught

11. Never leave the client alone to prevent injury from falls

12. Observe the client for swallowing reflexes. If not present, keep the client in a side lying position to prevent the tongue falling back and obstructing the airway.

13. Quickly observe the functioning of all devices and make sure they are in its functioning order, e.g. the drainage tubes are connected with the drainage bottle

14. Check the doctors orders for other instructions and treatment
15. Care of the client who is under the effect of anesthesia—client needs close and diligent observation until the client fully recover from anesthesia
16. Observe for vital sings, blood pressure, pulse rate, respiration rate, skin color, skin temperature
17. Intake and output—intravenous fluids, oral fluids taken by the client, naso-gastric aspiration, wound drainage, blood loss.
18. Abdominal girth in clients with abdominal distension
19. Urine output—time and amount
20. Bowel movements
21. Signs of hypo/hypervolemia
22. Any breathing difficulties
23. Pain over the calf muscles
24. Operation site for bleeding, drainage
25. Any specific observation told by surgeon

Common Management of Postoperative Complications

1. Shock
2. Hemorrhage
3. Wound infection
4. Respiratory complications
5. Thrombophlebitis
6. GI complications—vomiting, thirst, disturbance of metabolism, hiccup
7. Urinary complications—difficulty in micturation.

Postoperative Health Teaching

1. Maintenance of personal hygiene
2. Diet that is allowed for client, any control of the diet
3. Ambulation: Activities that are permitted, as well as restricted
4. Any adjustments to be made in the occupation of the client
5. Any drugs to be taken postoperatively, the side effects and precautions

6. Date on which the client may resume duty
7. Further treatment may be needed

Nursing care of the client during all phases of the surgical experience needs to be continuous and integrated. She takes all measures to prevent complications.

OPD Surgical Client

1. Review all instructions in the preoperative and postoperative regimen
2. Confirm place and time of surgery, including when to arrive
3. Ask client to pay the charges of surgery/procedure
4. Take the informed consent
5. Discuss what to wear
6. Explain a need for a responsible adult to drive or accompany the client home
7. Discuss discharge criteria and how long the client should expect to stay postoperatively
8. Discuss medications, including specific preoperative medications and the clients current medication regimen.
9. Communicate by telephone the evening before surgery to confirm time of surgery and arrival time.

Immediate Postanesthetic Phase

1. Adequacy of airway
2. Oxygen saturation
3. Adequacy of ventilation—respiratory rate, rhythm, and depth, use of accessory muscles, breath sounds
4. Cardiovascular status—heart rate and rhythm, peripheral pulse amplitude and equality, blood pressure, capillary filling
5. Level of consciousness—not responding, arousals with verbal stimuli, fully awake, oriented to time, person, and place
6. Presence of protective reflexes (e.g. gag, cough)
7. Activity, ability to move extremities
8. Skin color (pink, pale, blotchy, cyanotic, jaundiced)

9. Fluid status—intake and output, status of IV infusions (type of fluid, rate, amount in container, patency of tubing) signs of dehydration or fluid overload
10. Condition of operative site
11. Status of dressing
12. Drainage (amount, type, and color)
13. Patency of and character and amount of drainage from catheters, tubes, and drains
14. Discomfort (pain, location, and severity, nausea, vomiting safety (that is necessary for side rails, call bell within reach)

Chapter 17

Skin Preparation for Surgery

Definition

Skin preparation is a preoperative procedure performed to decontaminate and reduce the number of organisms on skin to eliminate the transference of such organisms into the incision site.

Purposes

1. To remove hair from well defined skin area
2. To prevent wound infection postoperatively
3. To prepare the part for surgery

Articles

1. Razor
2. New blade
3. Soap
4. Bowel with water
5. Rag pieces/paper tissue
6. Kidney basin
7. Mackintosh/waterproof pad
8. Basin with water
9. Sponge towel
10. Bath towel
11. Duster
12. Clean gloves
13. Scissors

Procedure

Preliminary Assessment

1. Inspect general condition of skin for any lesions, irritation
2. Hair removal upon site of incision, nature of surgery and physicians order carried out
3. Wash hands
4. Provide privacy by closing door or pulling screen
5. Position client comfortably with surgical site accessible so nurse has easy access to reach area
6. Don clean gloves
7. Remove hair—wet shave place towel/waterproof pad to prevent soiling bed linen
8. Shave small area at a time. Hold razor at 45° angle and shave in the direction of hair growth. Use short gentle strokes. So that it minimizes chances of cutting skin, and prevents pulling of hair
9. Rinse razor in basin of water as soap and hair accumulate on the blade, discard blades
10. Use wash cloth and warm water to rinse away remaining hair and soap solution from skin.
11. Inform client that procedure is completed

After Procedure

12. Clean and dispose articles
13. Wash hands
14. Record procedure in nurses notes
15. Report any skin alteration/cuts in skin to surgeon

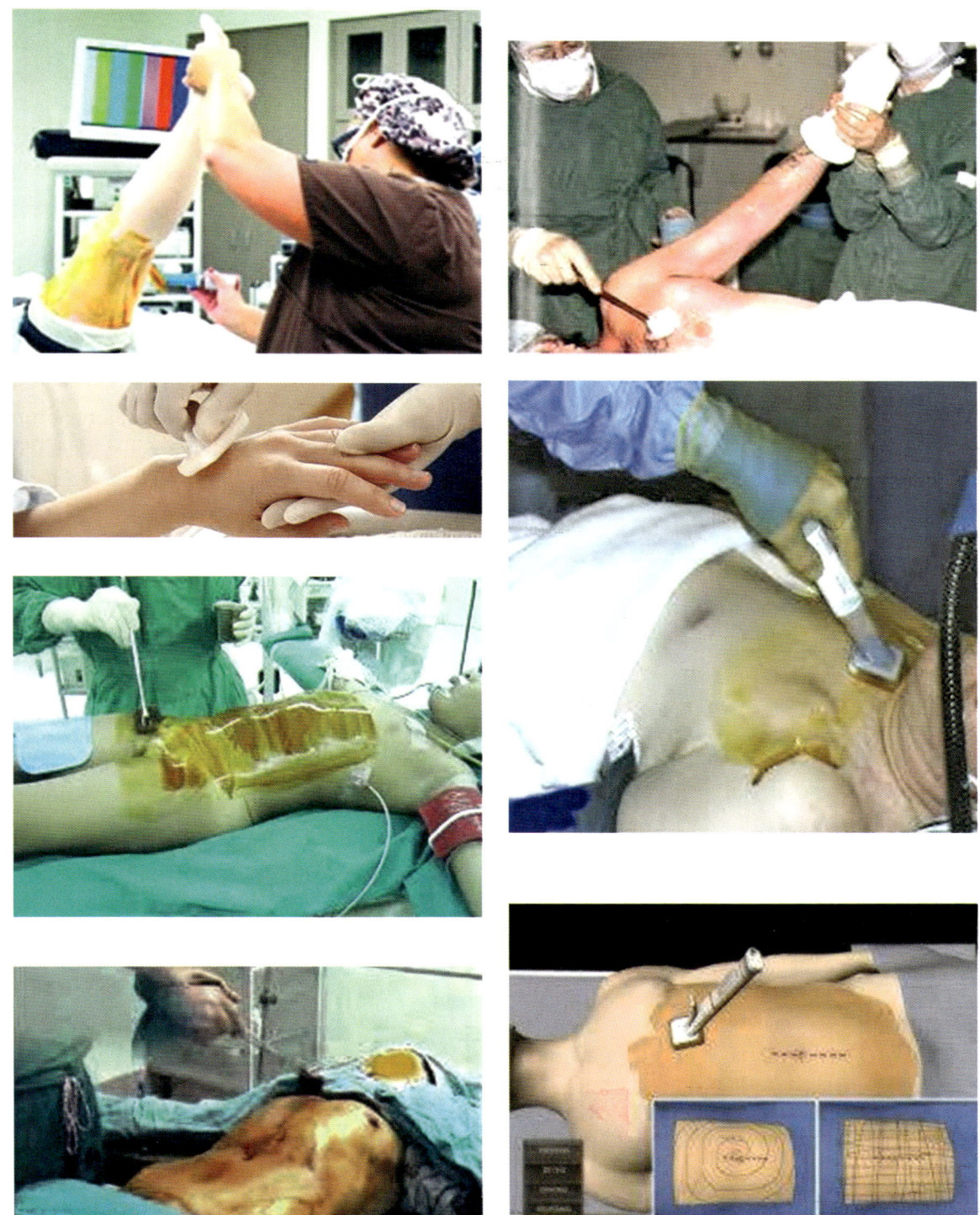

Fig. 17.1: Skin preparation before surgical procedure (as per site of operation skin is prepared)

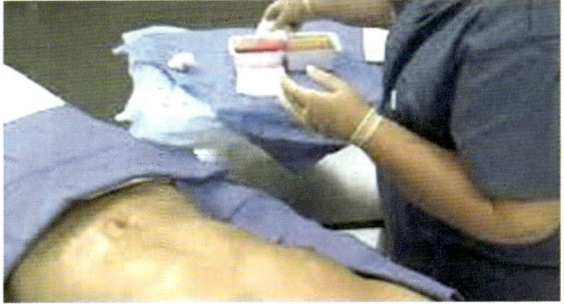

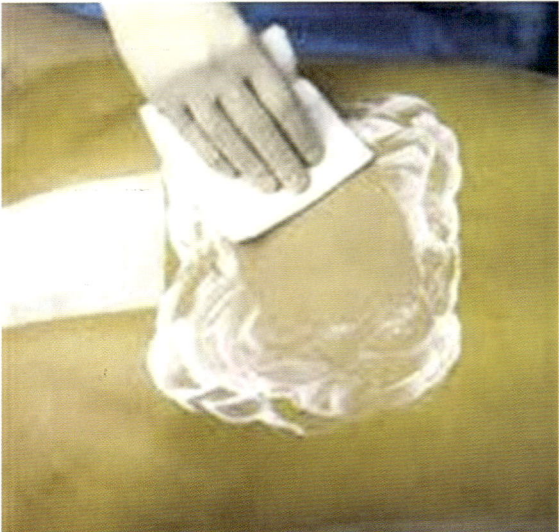

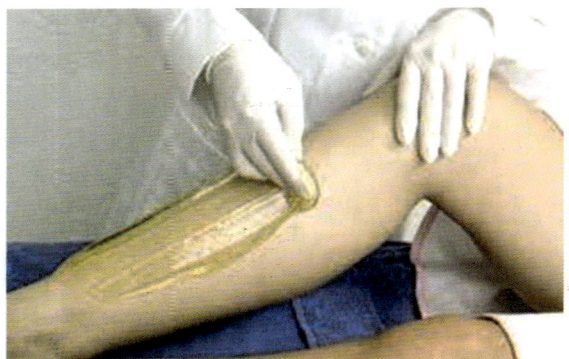

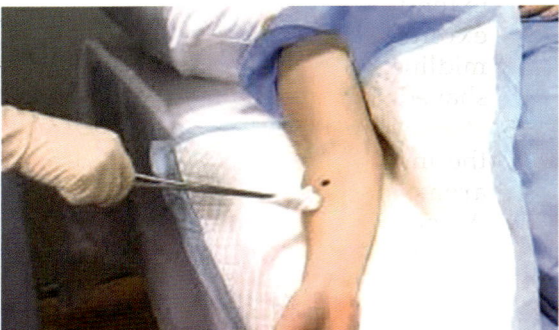

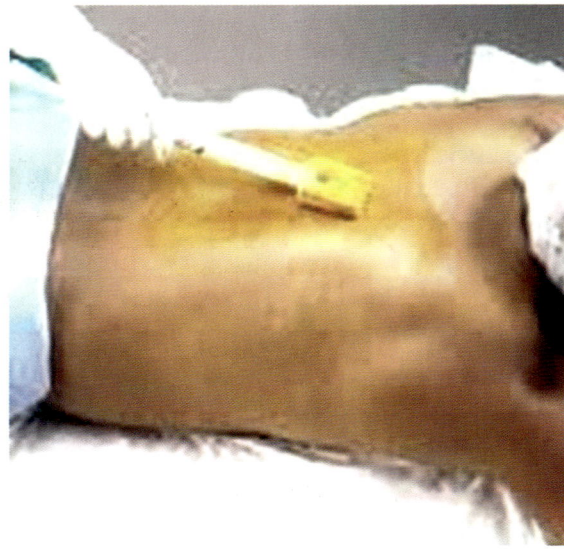

Fig. 17.2: Skin preparation before surgery

Site of Surgical Preparation

1. *Head and neck:* The site extends from above the eyebrows over the top of the head and includes the ears and both anterior and posterior areas of the neck and face. In female face is not shaved.

2. *Lateral neck:* Clean and external auditory canal with a cotton swab. Anteriorly, prepare the side of the face from above the ear to the upper thorax to just below the clavicle. Posteriorly prepare from neck to the spine including the area above the scapula.

3. *Chest surgery:* The site extends from the neck to the umbilicus and to the lateral midline.

4. *Abdominal surgery:* The preparation site extends from axilla to the mid thigh extending bilaterally to the lateral midline. All visible pubic hair should be shaved.

5. *Perineal surgery:* Shaves pubic hair and the inner thighs to the mid thigh. The areas starts above the pubic bone Anteriorly and extends beyond the anus posteriorly.

6. *Lumbar spine surgery:* Shave entire back including shoulders and neck to hairline and down to knees including both axilla.

7. *Rectal surgery:* Shaves buttocks from iliac crest down to the upper third of the thighs including the anal region. The area extends to the mid line on each side.

8. *Flank surgery:* Extends anteriorly from the axilla down to the upper thigh including external genital area. Posteriorly the area extends form mid scapular to the mid gluteal regions.

9. *Hand and forearm surgery:* The area includes the full circumference of the affected hand from axilla to the fingertips.

10. *Lower extremity surgery:* The area includes the area from umbilicus anteriorly including the entire leg, toes, and foot of the affected leg and posteriorly from top of buttocks to the heel.

11. *Lower leg surgery:* The area to be prepared includes the circumference of the entire leg from mid thigh to toes of the affected leg.

Note: Sometimes the site for preparation may vary according to the surgeon's preference.

Chapter 18

Preparation of Operation Theater Trolley

Definition

Keeping the operating room ready and available for carrying out surgical procedure.

Purposes

1. To ensure that appropriate equipment and machinery are available in working condition
2. To clean required equipment and medicines
3. To disinfect room, and work surfaces
4. To collect necessary supplies of sterile and other terms

Articles

1. Operating room table and accessories like lights, cautery, sponge rack, etc.
2. Instrument trolleys
3. Articles required for positioning client
4. Sterile linen
5. Instrument sets
6. Cleaning solutions
7. Waste disposal; containers

Procedure

1. Acquire information about the surgery to be carried out for quick and easy preparation of operating room
2. Assemble necessary equipment and machines to save time and energy and provide an organized approach to task

3. Disinfect room, work surfaces, walls and floor including equipment and machines. Carbolise the surfaces and equipment after wet washing to maintain sterile field.
4. Collect sterile linen and instrument set
5. Ensure that scrub room is ready with soap, running water and sterile brush
6. Ensure that air-conditioning, lighting and cautery machine for proper functioning
7. Connect suction apparatus to electric source and check central suction equipment.
8. Receive client to operating room
9. All personnel working in the operation theater use special dresses and shoes which are kept for use only for the time of theater work.
10. Anyone entering inside the theater after carbonizing, should wear cap and mask along with the theater gown.

STERILE TECHNIQUE OF DRAPING TROLLEY

Definition

Arranging appropriate sterile linen, instruments and supplies on designated trolleys for carrying out surgical operation, using aseptic technique.

Purposes

1. To create a sterile field for carrying out surgical operation

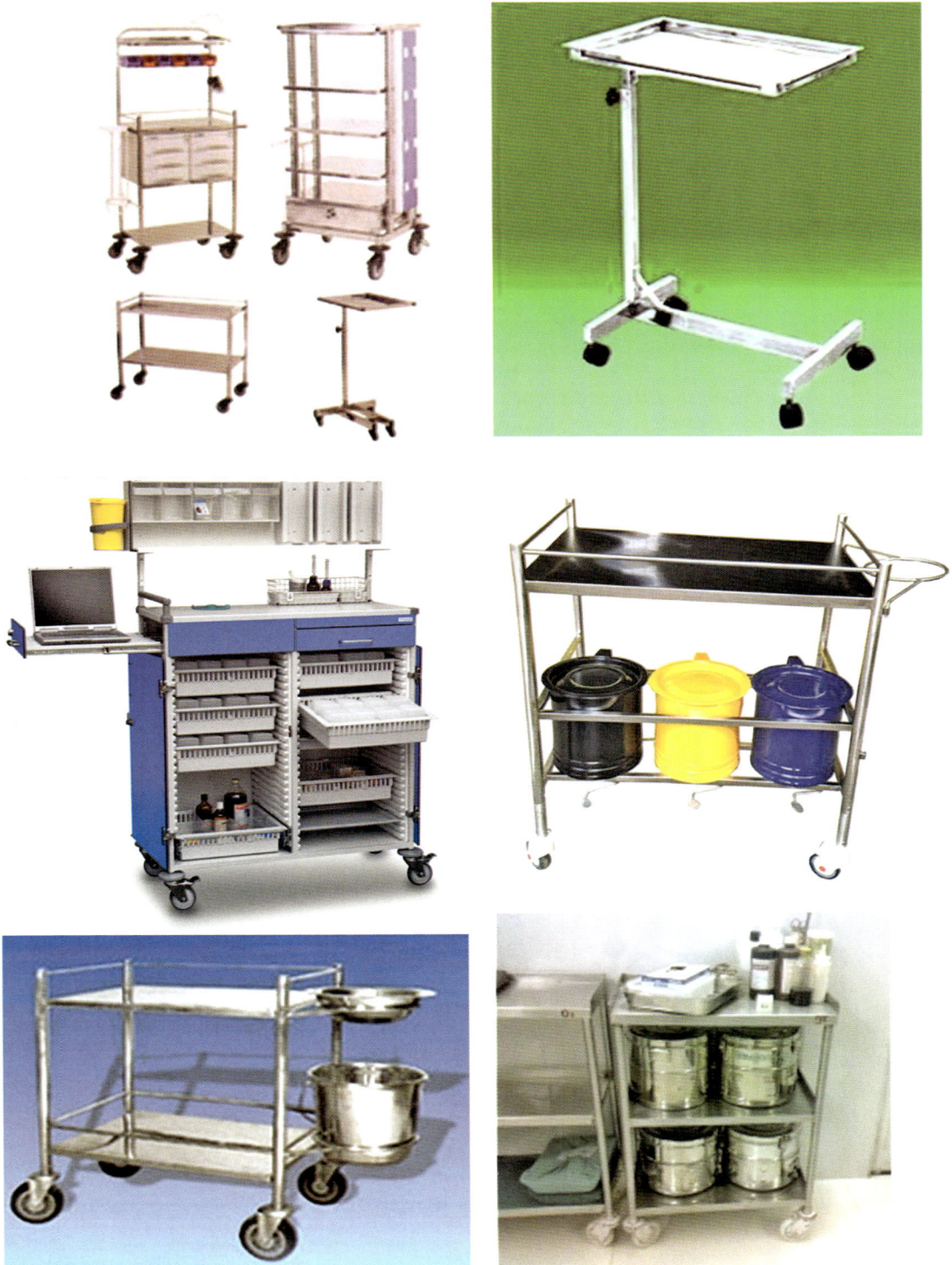

Fig. 18.1: Different types of operation theater trolleys

2. To ensure successful barrier against bacterial invasion of surgical wound

Articles

1. Instrument trolleys
2. Mayo stand
3. Basin stand
4. Square trolley

Procedure

1. Scrub nurse puts on sterile cap, mask, gown and gloves after scrubbing her hands.
2. Check outer labels of all sterile linen bundles and instrument sets to ensure that correct instrument sets are opened.
3. Follow principles of asepsis while sterile packs are opened, maintain sterile field.
4. Circulating nurse, opens the sterile drum and handover the sterile towel with the transfer forceps to the scrubbed nurse.
5. Scrubbed nurse spreads the towel carefully on the trolley without touching unsterile area.
6. Drape distal end of trolley first, then proximal
7. The circulating nurse opens the sterile pack using transfer forceps and scrub nurse removes the instrument tray and instrument from the sterile pack and gently places on instrument trolley.
8. Arrange instruments neatly according to the order of use.
9. Circulating nurse pours sterile saline in sterile basin which is placed in basin stand.
10. Discard unnecessary wraps and foils from sterile field.
11. Discard any contaminated drapes/ instruments and substitute with sterile ones. A sterile work area promotes proper aseptic technique.
12. After arranging, cover the trolley with a sterile towel till it is taken over for surgery

STERILE TECHNIQUE OF DRAPING CLIENT

Definition

Receiving the preoperative client on the theater table, and replacing clients linen with sterile, theater linen, exposing operative site for preoperative skin cleaning and placing sterile mackintosh and towels for barricading operative site from surrounding areas.

Purposes

1. To create a sterile field for carrying out surgical operation
2. To ensure successful barrier against bacterial invasion of surgical wound
3. To prevent contamination of operative site with unprepared skin surfaces

Articles

1. Sterile bed linen
2. Big and small mackintosh
3. Surgical towels
4. Towel clips

Procedure

1. Transfer the client to theater table.
2. Replace clients linen with sterile linen so that sterile field is maintained.
3. Expose operative site while adequately covering other areas.
4. Assist surgeon to clean the site with bacteriological solution.
5. Offer sterile, towels and towel clip to surgeon and assist in draping operative site
6. Drape client acceding to nature, type of surgery and incision.
7. Secure towel clips at each corner, viz above, below and sides of operative site.
8. Assist surgeon to app "Opsite" evenly without air pockets, soon after cleaning and drying operative site.

APPLYING MASK AND STERILE GOWN

Definition

This procedure involves wearing of a mask and a specially stitched gown in the operation theater to maintain asepsis.

And to protect the nurse from contaminating herself and others around her.

Purposes

1. To prevent dispersal of droplets from wearer to environment and client
2. To prevent contamination of sterile field
3. To enhance easy handling of sterile equipment.

Procedure

1. After performing surgical hand washing take the sterile mask handed to you by circulating nurse. Hold it by top two strings, keeping top edge above bridge of nose.
2. Tie both top strings at back of head above ears
3. Tie the two lower strings snugly around neck well under the chin
4. Ensure proper fitting

Gowning

1. Grasp the sterile gown at the crease near the neck, hold it away from yourself and permit it to unfold freely without touching anything including the uniform. To prevent gown from becoming unsterile.
2. Hold the gown at the shoulder level from inside and put each hand directly into the armhole, and protect the outer portion of gown from contamination.
3. Extend the arms and hold hand upward at shoulder level while putting through the armhole.
4. The circulating nurse pulls back the gown from inside. So that the upper limbs go into the sleeves. The circulating nurse ties the gown from the back.

5. The waist ties are loosened by the scrub nurse and flap is brought around the waist by the use of cheatle forceps held by the circulating nurse and is tied. The waist flap cover the back, preventing contamination of the area when turning around.

Removing of the Gown

1. Untie strings at the back of the gown. Remove gown, folding inside out to cover outside of gown.
2. Dispose gown into designated receptacle

Removing of the Mask

1. Wash hands, untie lower strings first, then the top stings and pull mask away from face.
2. Hold mask by strings and discard into designated receptacle.

PERFORMING STERILE GLOVING

Definition

Gloving is defined as the donning of a pair of sterile gloves to protect ones own hands from pathogenic microorganisms' and to avoid contamination of a sterile area by hand.

Purposes

1. To protect the nurse from pathogenic microorganisms
2. To handle sterile articles without contaminating

Procedure

1. Perform thorough surgical hand wash and dry hands using sterile towel
2. The circulating nurse removes the outer glove package by carefully separating and peeling apart the sides. Scrubbed nurse pulls out the inner gloves pack taking care not to touch the outer one. This prevents inner glove package from accidentally opening and touching contaminated objects.

3. Grasp inner package and lay it on clean, flat surface just above waist level. Open package, keeping gloves on wrappers inside surface.
4. If gloves are not pre-powdered, take packet of powder and apply lightly to hands over sink or waste basket.
5. Identify right and left give. Each glove has a cuff of approximately 5 cm (2 inches) wide. Glove dominant hand first.
6. With thumb and first two fingers of non-dominant hand, grasp edge of cuff of glove of dominant hand. Touch only the inside surface of gloves.
7. Carefully pull glove over dominant hand making sure the thumb and fingers fit into the proper spaces of the glove.
8. Slip in the fingers of the gloved dominant hand under the cuff of the other glove.

Keep thumb of gloved dominant hand abducted back to avoid touching of exposed non-gloved hand.

9. Carefully slip the glove onto your non-dominant hand making sure that the fingers slip into the proper spaces.
10. With gloved hands, interlock fingers to fit gloves onto each fingers.

Removal of Gloves

1. Remove the first glove by gasping it on its palmer surface taking care to avoid touching wrist.
2. Pull the first glove completely off by inverting or rolling the glove inside out. Discard in receptacle.
3. Wash hands.

Chapter 19

Sterile Technique

DEFINITION

An object is sterile only when it is free of all microorganisms, e.g. before an operating room procedure, the 'scrub' nurse generally puts on a mask and cap, performs a surgical hand scrub, and then do a sterile gown and gloves.

Purpose

To ensure that sterile items remain sterile.

Sterile field is a microorganism-free area.

Surgical asepsis or sterile technique—refers to those practices that keep an area or object free of all microorganisms; it includes practices that destroy all microorganisms and spores (microscopic, Dorman structures formed by some pathogens that are very hardy and often survive common cleaning technique surgical asepsis is used for all procedures involving the sterile areas of the body.

1. All objects used in a sterile field must be sterile. All articles are sterilized appropriately by dry or moist heat, chemicals, or radiation before use.
2. Always check a package containing a sterile object for intactness, dress, and expiration date.
3. Sterile articles can be stored for only a prescribed time, after that, they are considered un-sterile.
4. Any package we storage areas should be clean, dry, off the floor, and away from sinks.
5. Sterile object becomes un-sterile when touched by un-sterile objects.
6. Whenever the sterility of an object is questionable, assume the article is un-sterile.
7. Sterile items that are out of vision or below the waist or table level are considered un-sterile
8. Only the front part of a sterile gown, from shoulder to waist and the cuff of the sleeves to 2 inches above the elbows are considered sterile.
9. When working over a sterile field, keep talking to a minimum.
10. Wear a surgical caps in operating rooms
11. Unless gloves are worn, always hold wet forceps with the tips below the handles. When he tips are held higher than he handles. Fluids can flow onto he handle and become contaminated by the hands. When the forceps are again pointed downward, the contaminated fluid flows back down and contaminates the tips.
12. During a surgical hand wash, hold the hands higher than to elbows to prevent contaminates from the forearms from reaching the hands.
13. Any article that falls outside the edges of a sterile field is considered un-sterile.

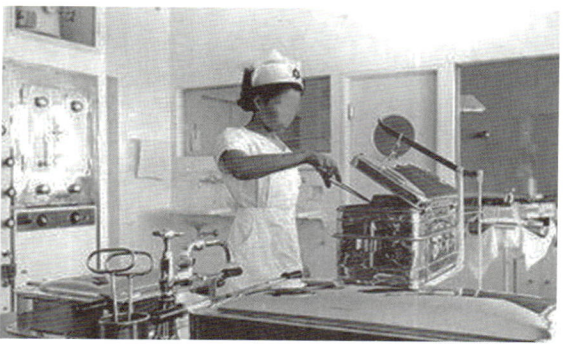
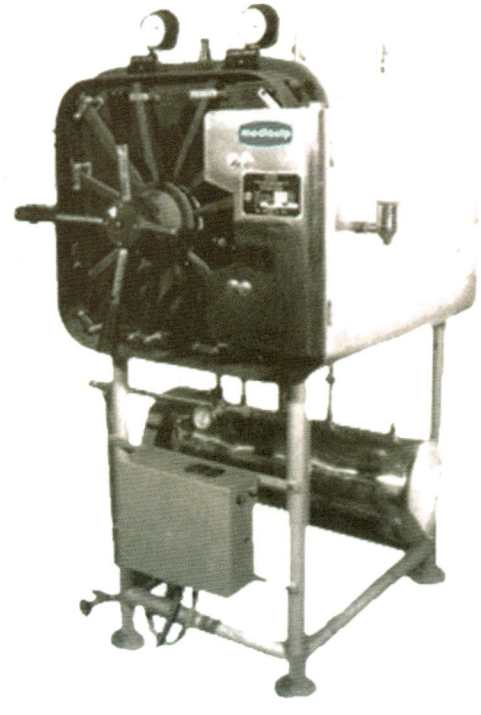
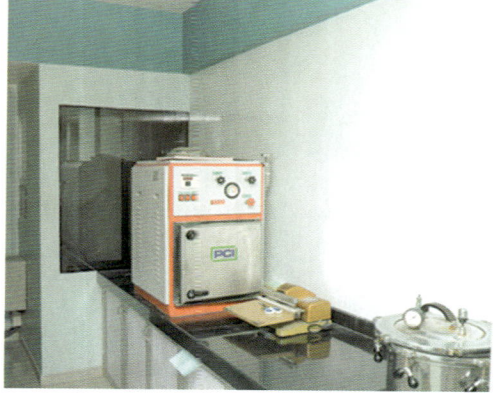
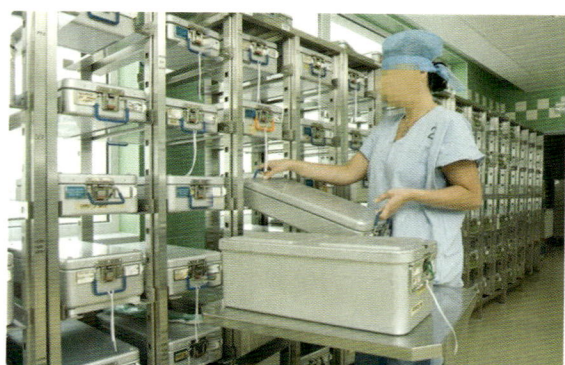
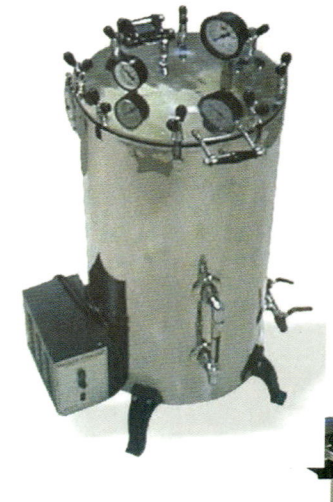
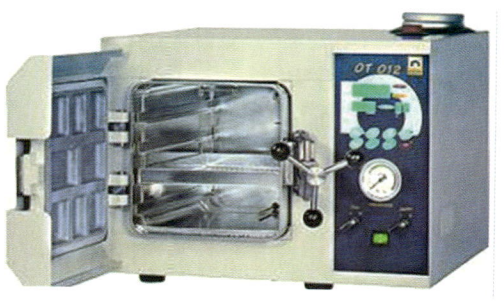
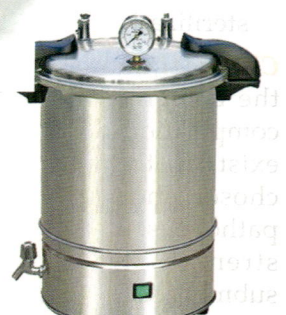

Fig. 19.1: Sterilization, autoclaving technique of surgical articles and instruments

14. Prior to a surgical aseptic procedure, cleanse the hands to reduce the number of microorganisms on them.

15. Consciousness, alertness, and honesty are essential qualities in maintaining surgical asepsis.

16. Do not set up a sterile field ahead of time for future use.

The first links in the chain of infection, the etiologic agent and the reservoir, are interrupted by the use of antiseptic and disinfectants and by sterilization.

STERILIZATION

Sterilization is a process that destroys all microorganisms, including spores and viruses. For commonly used methods of sterilization is moist heat, gas, boiling water, and radiation.

1. *Moist heat:* To sterilize with moist heat (such as with an autoclave) steam under pressure is used because it attains temperatures higher than the boiling point

2. *Gas:* Ethylene oxide gas destroys microorganisms by interfering with their metabolic process. It is effective against spores. Its advantages are good penetrating and effectiveness for heat sensitive items. Its major disadvantage is toxicity to humans.

3. *Boiling water:* This is most practical and inexpensive method for sterilizing in the home.

4. *Radiation:* Both ionizing and non ionizing radiations are used for disinfection and sterilization.

Chemical disinfection: Acts by coagulating the bacterial protein or by changing the composition of protein so that it no longer exists in the same form. The disinfectant chosen should be efficient to destroy the pathogens. They should be used in correct strength. The articles should be fully submerged in it.

They are applied for a sufficient length of time. They should not be injurious to the skin and articles. The article should be thoroughly cleaned and dried before immersing in the disinfectant to remain free from organic material which will protect the bacteria against the action of disinfectants. The disinfectant should be inexpensive. Instruments soaked in disinfectants must be adequately rinsed with sterile water before being used.

Autoclaving Steam under Pressure

Autoclaving is a method of sterilization by steam under pressure. It is to most widely used, economical and one of the most effective methods of destroying microorganisms. This method uses temperature, pressure and humidity to destroy all types of microorganisms, including spore forming. The steam under pressure maintains the necessary high temperature and it allows rapid penetration of articles packed in it.

For effective sterilization autoclaving is done at 15 lbs per square inch pressure and 121°C temperature for at least 20 minutes.

Autoclaving is used to sterilize all kinds of articles except those which are destroyed by high temperature and steam, e.g. plastic and rubber goods.

Important Points to Consider

1. All the air from the inner chamber must be driven out and replaced by steam otherwise the desired temperature of 121°C at 15 lbs/inch of pressure would not be reached

2. The packed material and articles therein for sterilization should be packed loosely to allow penetration of the steam.

3. The packed material should not be very large and should be well separated to allow the circulation of steam.

4. The pressure is maintained at 15 lbs per square inch and the thermometer reads at least 121°C without downward fluctuations for at least 20 minutes.

5. The article should be left in the autoclave for a short time after the procedure is over in order to dry materials.
6. *Fumigation or gas sterilization*
7. Total surface exposure to formaldehyde gas under conditions of controlled humidity temperature and time exposure will destroy all vegetative forms of bacteria, viruses and most of the spores. The best results can be obtained with high concentration of gas, humidity above 60 and temperature of not les than 18°C. The exposure time varies from one to 16 hours. The agents commonly used for the fumigation are formalin tablets, ethylene oxide liquids, etc.
8. *Fumigation with sulphur*
9. The room should be filled with steam by a kettle of water in the room as the sulphur fumes act better on a damp place. A small room of 100 square feet requires about 220 gms of sulphur which is placed in earthen ware which stands in a large container with water. A little methylated spirit poured over the sulphur to ensure burning the sulphur completely. Lit fire to sulphur and close door. The rooms open after 24 hours. Effectiveness depends on gas concentration, temperature, time, humidity. All articles should be open for penetration of fumes.
10. *Fumigation with formalin*
11. Formalin is more efficacious as a surface disinfectant. For every 100 square feet of room space 140 grams of potassium permanganate crystal and 120 ml of formalin mix it and place temperature in a metal bowl. Heat produced by chemical action evaporates the formaldehyde. Room should be sealed for 12 to 14 hours. After that keep open.
12. It has a pungent smell and it irritant to eyes, skin and mucus membrane.

Chapter 20

Positioning Client for Surgery

Definition

Providing specific positions for clients undergoing surgery, which promote best visualization and accessibility to operative site and promote safety and comfort.

Purposes

1. To provide necessary accessibility and exposure for the site to be operated.
2. To facilitate administration of anesthesia and efficient monitoring.
3. To ensure safety for the client and prevent injury.
4. To promote normal circulatory and respiratory functions.
5. To provide correct skeletal alignment.
6. To prevent under pressure on muscles, nerves, skin over bony prominences and eyes.

Factors that Determine Position

1. The surgery to be performed
2. Types of anesthesia used
3. Age, size and physical condition of the client
4. Surgical approach

Articles

1. Head rest
2. Arm board
3. Sand bag
4. Pillows
5. Towel roll
6. Mackintosh
7. Straps
8. Stirrups
9. Drapes

Positions used in Surgery

Supine position used in abdominal operations, thoracic, abdominothoracic operation, operation of hip, lower extremities operation, for radical mastectomy (Fig. 20.1).

Other Common Position

Patient to check vitals, do physical examination, transporting helpless patient (from bed to structures, sutures to bed, wheelchair and vice versa) lifting, moving, mobilizing, supporting, for patient after anesthesia to prevent aspiration of saliva, mucus and blood, and different positions used in surgery like dorsal, lateral, laminectomy, lithotomic, Sims, supine, and Trendelenburg, etc.

Rose position/neck position: Thyroidectomy, tacheostomy, parathyroidectomy.

Leg exercise during surgery venous blood returns from the legs slows, in addition some surgical position decrease venous return. Thrombophlebitis and resultant emboli are

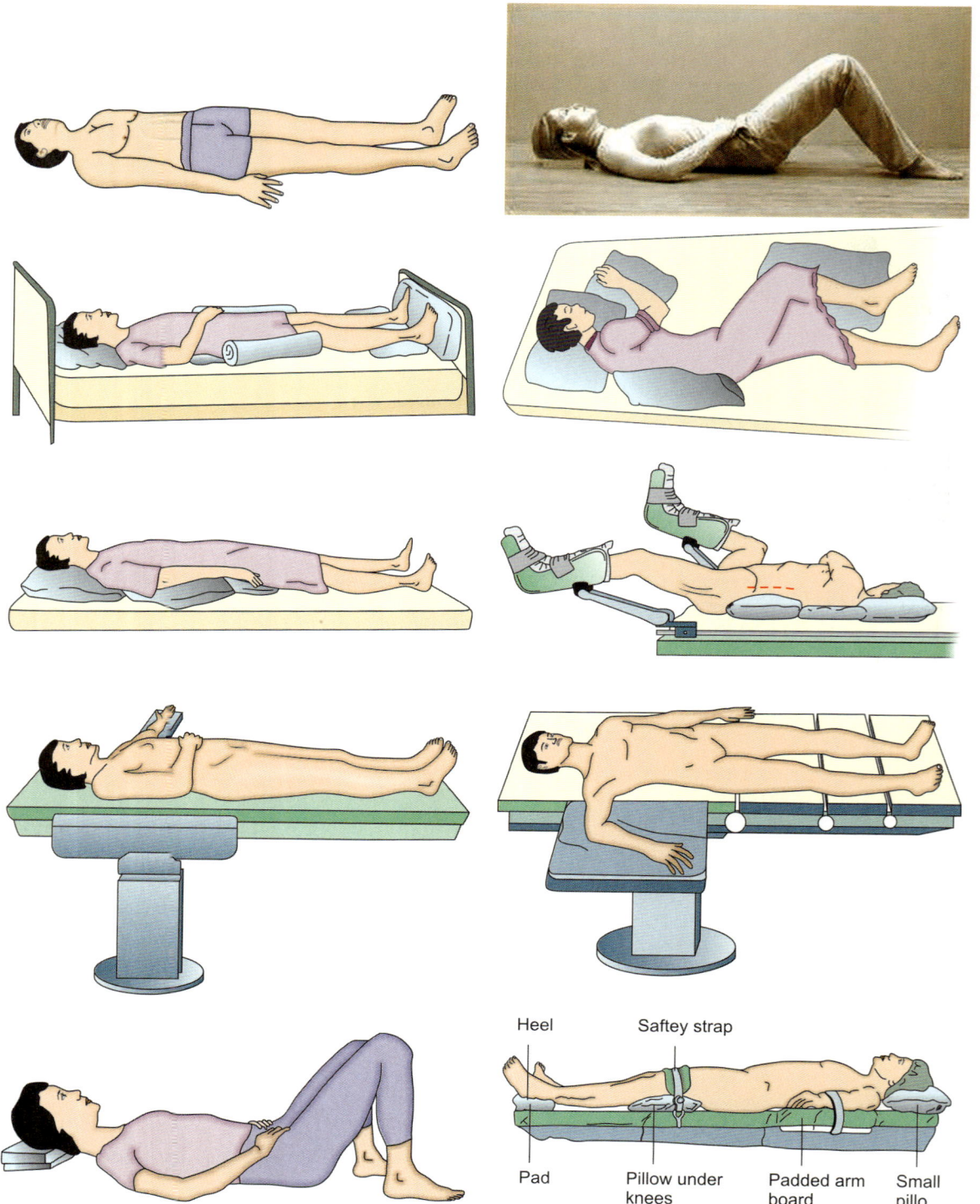

Fig. 20.1: Supine position as per site of procedure

Prone position: Thoracic/lumbar, laminectomy

Lithotomy position: Cystoscopy, operations of vagina, perineum and rectum

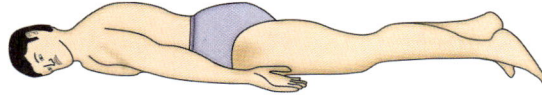

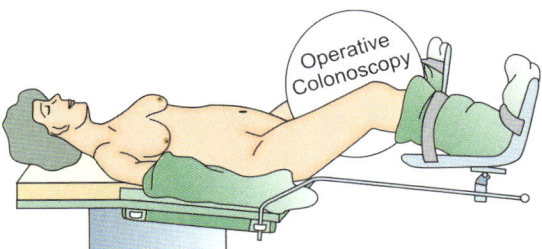
Operative Colonoscopy

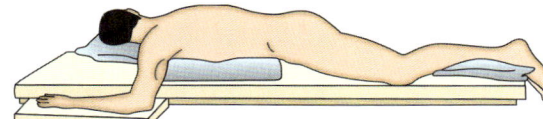

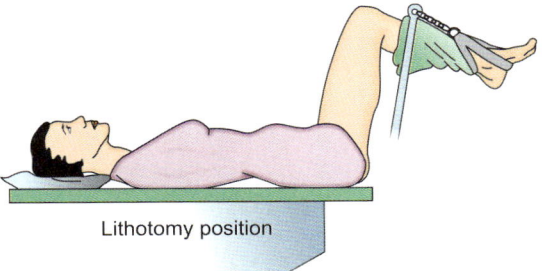
Lithotomy position

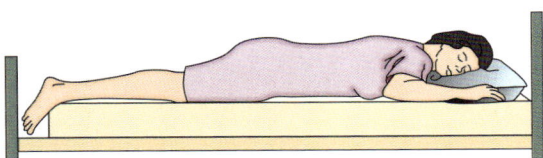

Head
Chin
Elbow
Chest
Reproductive organ
Knee
toes

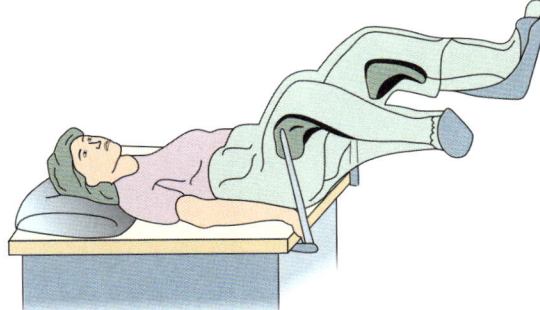

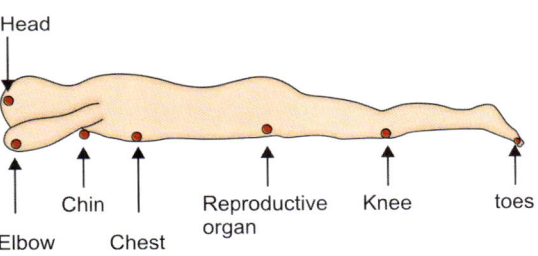

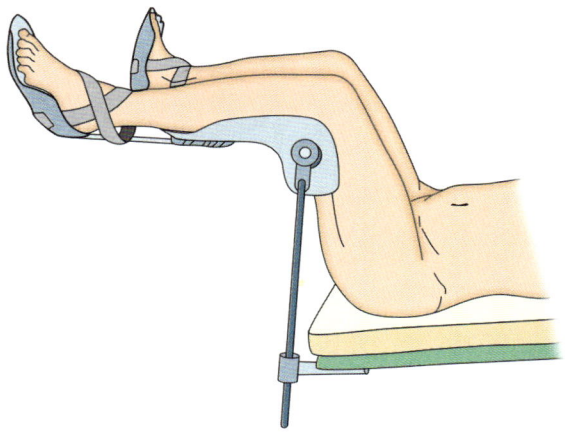

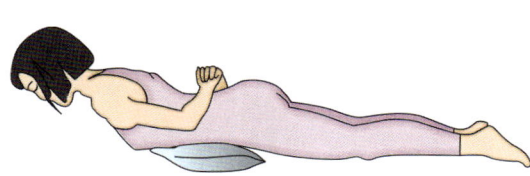

Fig. 20.2: Prone position

Fig. 20.3: Lithotomy position

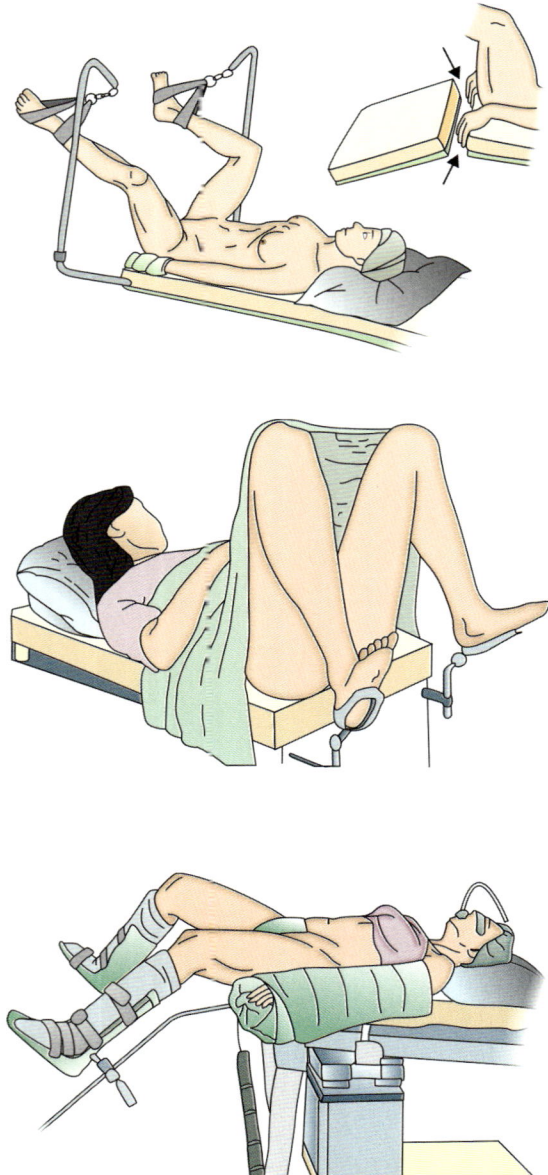

Fig. 20.4: Lithotomy position

potential complication from this circulation stasis in the leg. Leg exercise increase venous return through flexion and contraction of there quadriceps and gastrocnemius muscles. Leg exercises must be individualized to patients needs, physical condition, primary care provider, preference and facility protocol

Trendelenburg position: Operations on lower abdomen and pelvis

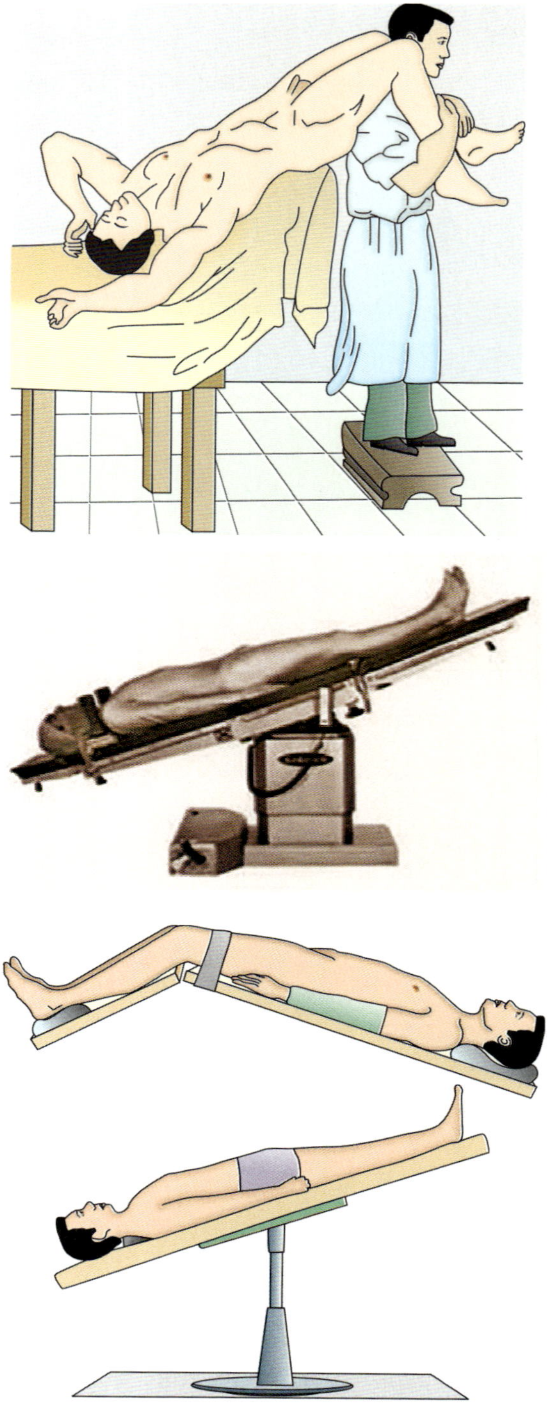

Fig. 20.5: Trendelenburg position

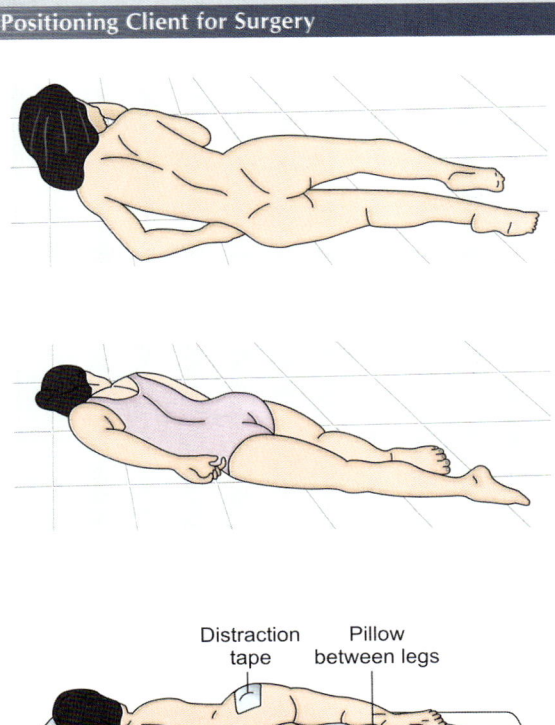

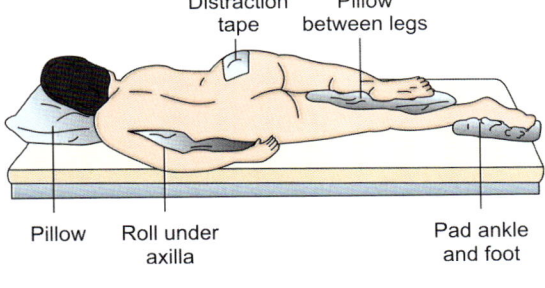

Distraction   Pillow
tape   between legs

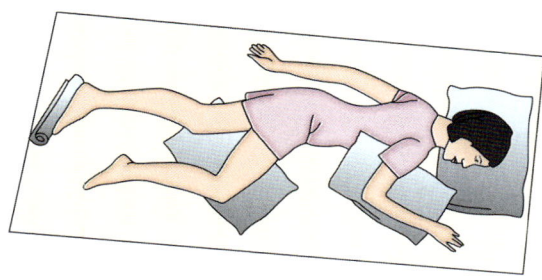

Pillow   Roll under   Pad ankle
         axilla   and foot

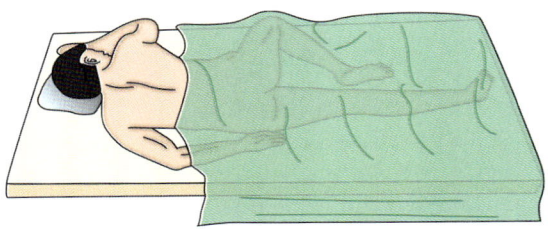

Fig. 20.6: Sims' position

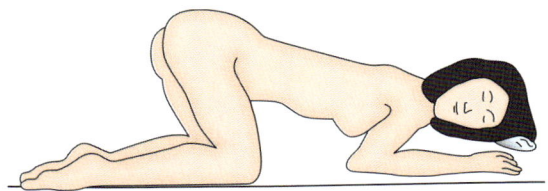

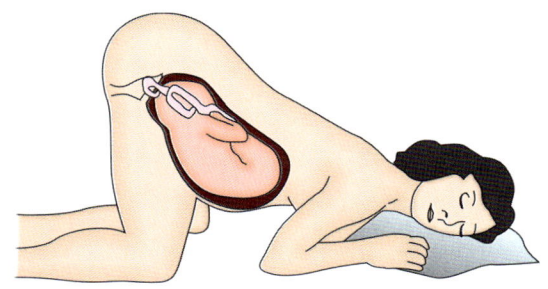

Fig. 20.7: Knee-chest position

Lateral position: Renal surgery

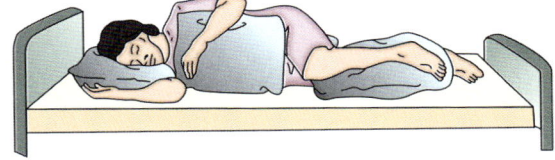

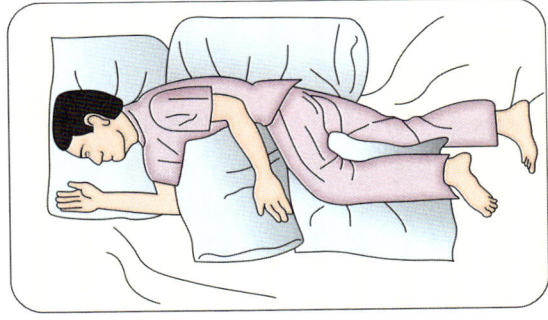

Fig. 20.8: Lateral position

Transferring a client using a powered full-body sling lift the client cannot bear any weight, use a powerful full body sling lift device to move them up in or out of bed, into and out of a chair and to a commode or stretcher. A full body sling is placed under

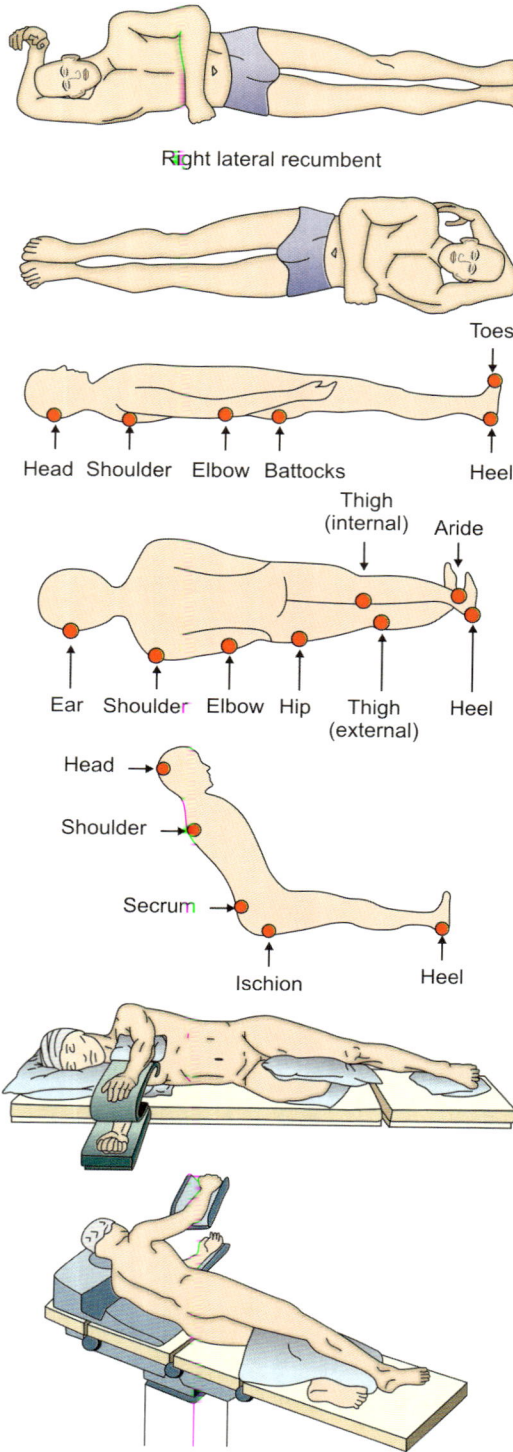

Right lateral recumbent

Head Shoulder Elbow Battocks   Heel

Ear Shoulder Elbow Hip Thigh (external) Heel

Thigh (internal)   Aride

Toes

Head

Shoulder

Secrum

Ischion   Heel

Fig. 20.9: Other surgical site position

the client's body including head and torso, and then the sling is attached to the lift. The device slowly lifts the client. Some devices can be lowered to the floor to pick up a patient who has fallen. These devices are available on portable bases and ceiling mounted tracks.

Note: Observe the client throughout the surgery. Protect any unprotected bony prominence or pressure point.

ASSISTING WITH POSTOPERATIVE EXERCISE

Definition

Exercises done by client independently or with assistance, to enhance a speedy recovery after surgery.

Exercise include:
1. Ambulation
2. Diaphragmatic breathing
3. Turning in bed
4. Leg exercise

Ambulation Exercise

Assisting a client to walk after a period of being immobile following surgery.

Purposes

1. To exercise muscles and joints for regaining strength
2. To increase clients sense of independence
3. To increase mobility
4. To prevent postoperative complications.

Procedure

1. Assess clients condition, vital signs and any contraindications.
2. Check the time when client received last dose of sedative drug.
3. Assess clients ability to walk.
4. Keep a foot stool beside bed if required keep a chair with back rest and extra pillow ready near the bed.
5. Make sure that the floor is clean and dry.
6. Explain procedure and purpose of ambulation.

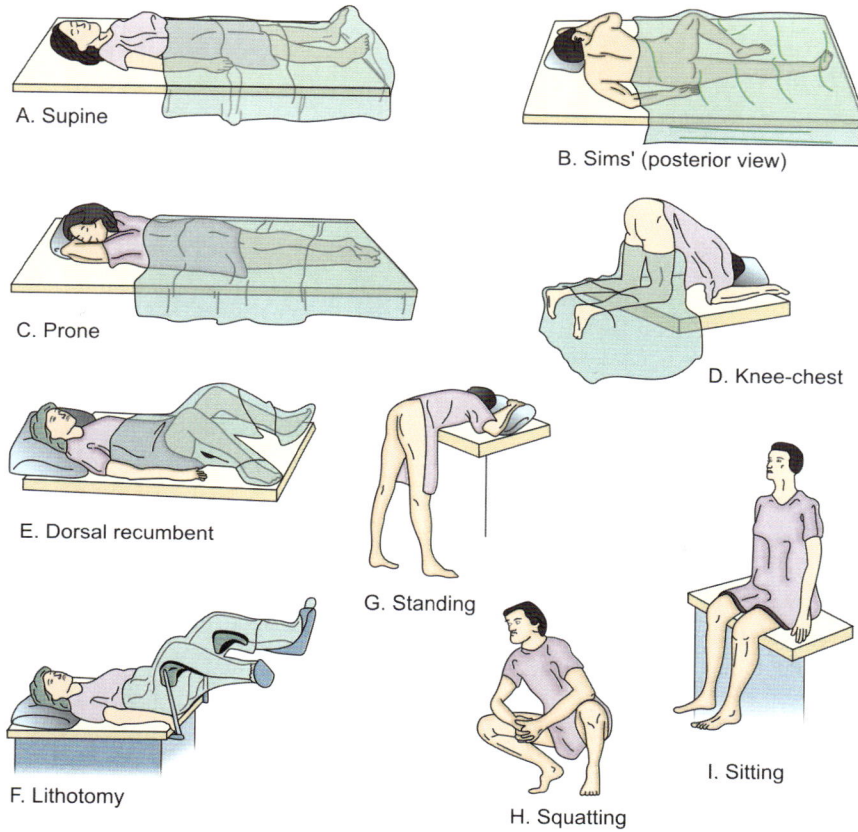

A. Supine

B. Sims' (posterior view)

C. Prone

D. Knee-chest

E. Dorsal recumbent

G. Standing

F. Lithotomy

H. Squatting

I. Sitting

Fig. 20.10

7. Ensure that client is adequately dressed and well groomed
8. Free all drain attached to bedside. Empty urobag, ensure that the drainage bag is held below hip level.

9. Raise head end to 40–60 degree and assist client to sit up. Brings client's legs to the edge of bed and allow feet to dangle (to prevent orthostatic hypotension)

Positions given according to the diseases condition

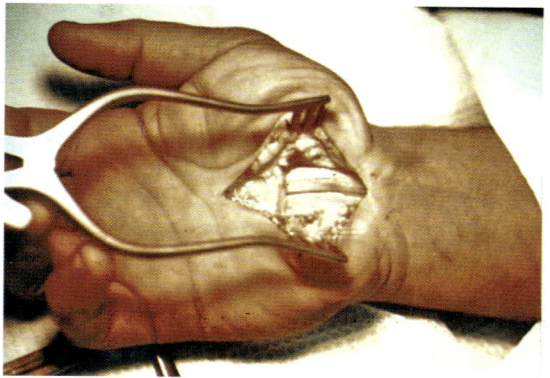

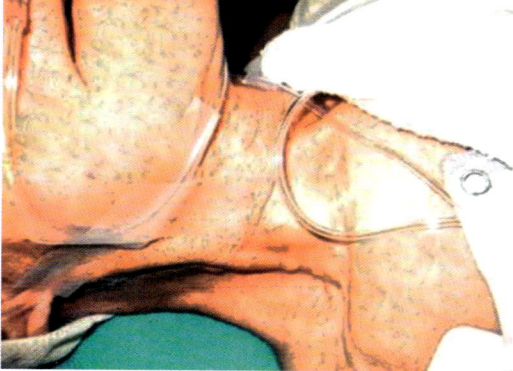

Fig. 20.11: Hand surgery position

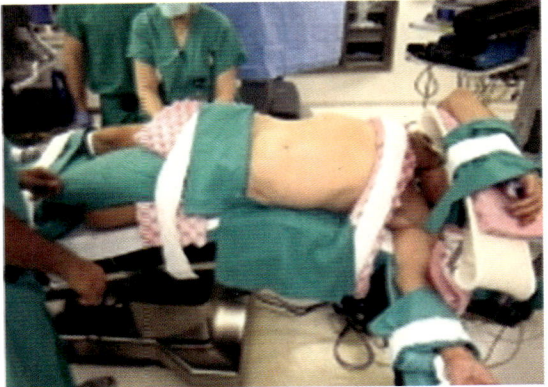

Fig. 20.12A: Positioning patient before surgery

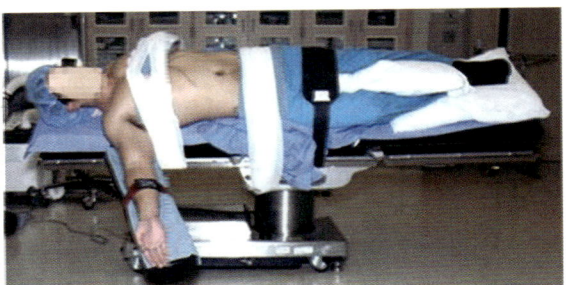

Fig. 20.12B: Position before surgery

10. Check for dizziness, drowsiness, pain. Ensure that client is able to tolerate ambulation.
11. Assist client to get out of bed slowly and to stand with head erect and back straight
12. Support client by either side by holding at inferior aspect and upper arms and assist him to walk with even gait to prevent accidental fall.
13. After walking, allow client to rest in chair for some time and then assist back to bed. Check vital signs and note untoward changes if any.
14. Connect the drains back in position and make client comfortable and leave the unit neat.
15. Record in clients chart the distance walked, duration of ambulation and clients response.

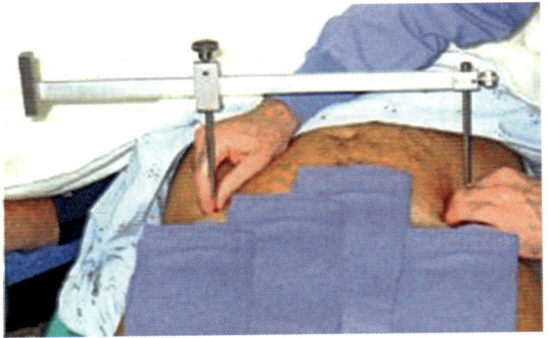

Fig. 20.13: Walsh pelvic level

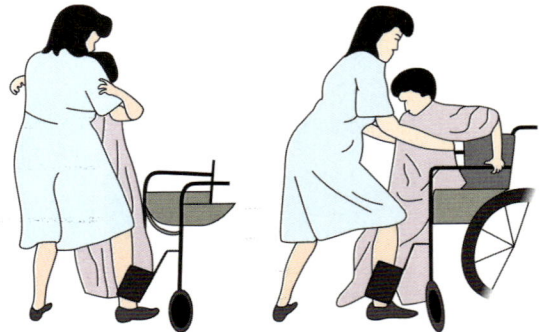

Fig. 20.14: Transfering client from wheel chair

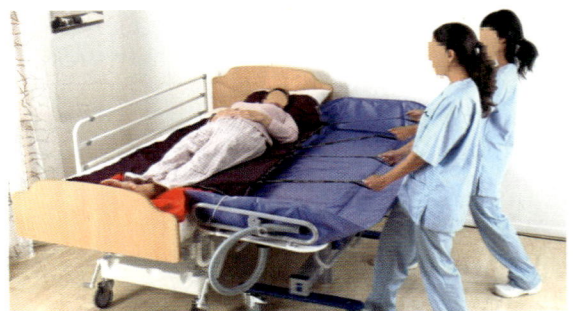

Fig. 20.15: Shifting technique

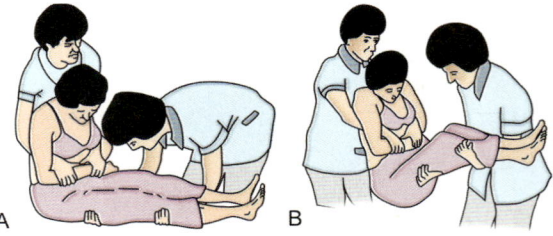

A   B

Fig. 20.16A and B: Lifting skills

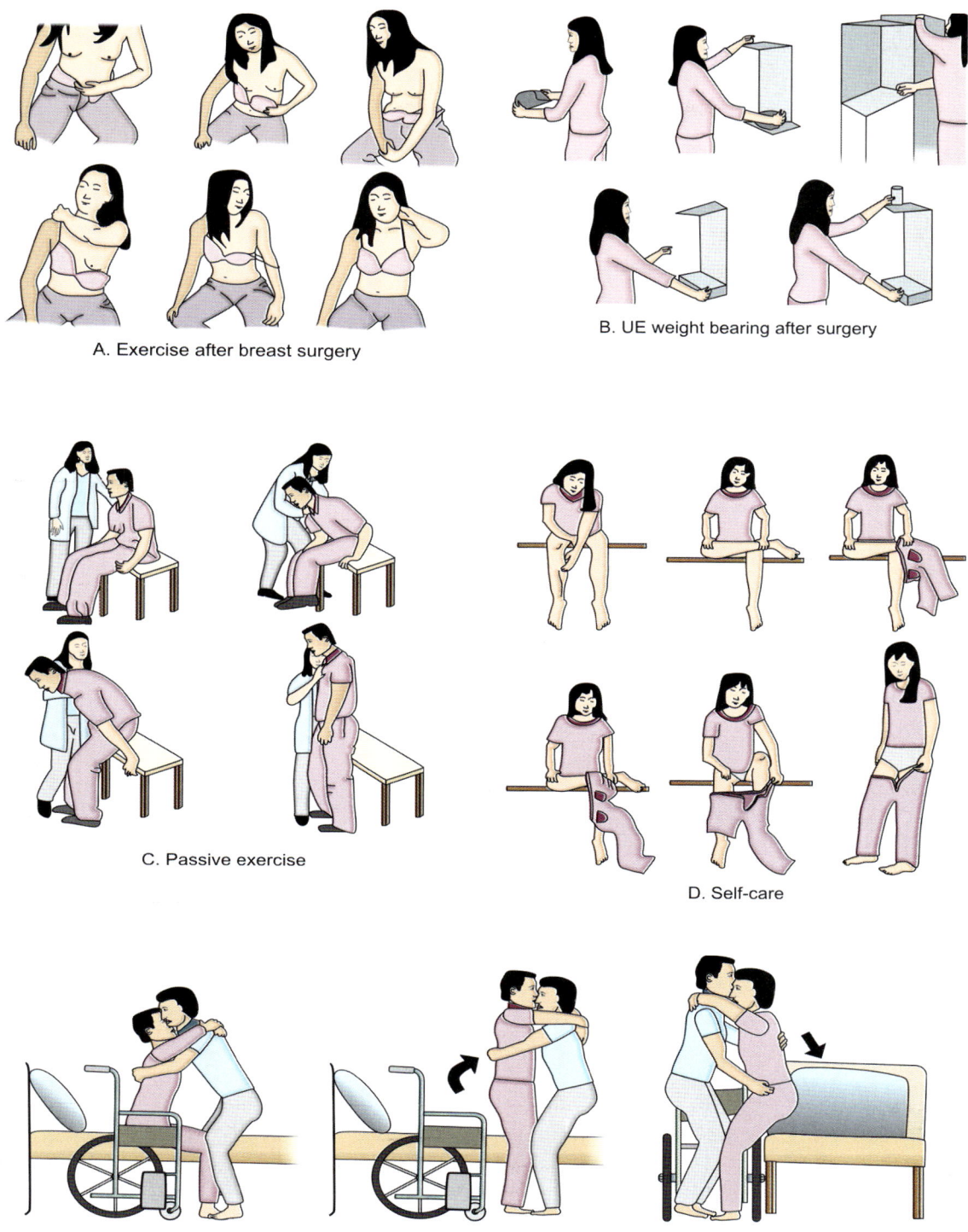

A. Exercise after breast surgery

B. UE weight bearing after surgery

C. Passive exercise

D. Self-care

E. Helping the patient to shift wheel chair

Fig. 20.17: Nursing role, exercise, transfering, helping the client to shift bed to wheel chair and vice versa

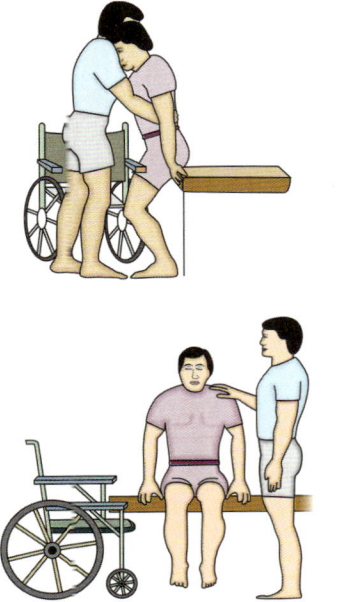

Fig. 20.18: Wheelchair to bed transfer

Types of Exercise

1. Diaphragmatic/deep breathing exercise
2. Controlled coughing
3. Turning exercise
4. Leg exercise

Documentation

The intraoperative nurse documents the per-operative plan of care including assessment, diagnosis, outcome, identification, planning, implementation, and evaluation.

The circulating nurse coordinates activities and manages clients care by continually assessing client safety, aseptic practice and the environment.

The scrub person's role is to assist the surgeons. They wear sterile gowns, gloves, caps, and eye protection. Their responsibilities include draping the client with sterile drapes and handling sterile instruments and supplies. The circulating nurse and scrub person are responsible for accounting of all sponges, needles, and instruments at the close of the surgery. This precaution avoids leaving any foreign bodies inside the client.

Traduction technique will teach the nurse how to transfer patient in safety manner keeping the body alignment which will save the time and energy and comfort to the patient.

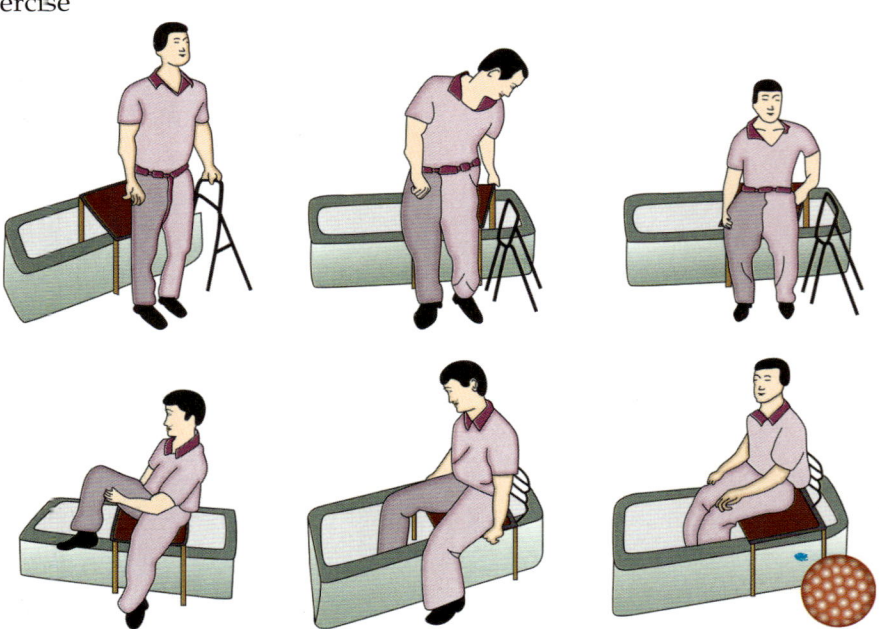

Fig. 20.19: Teaching client the right movements

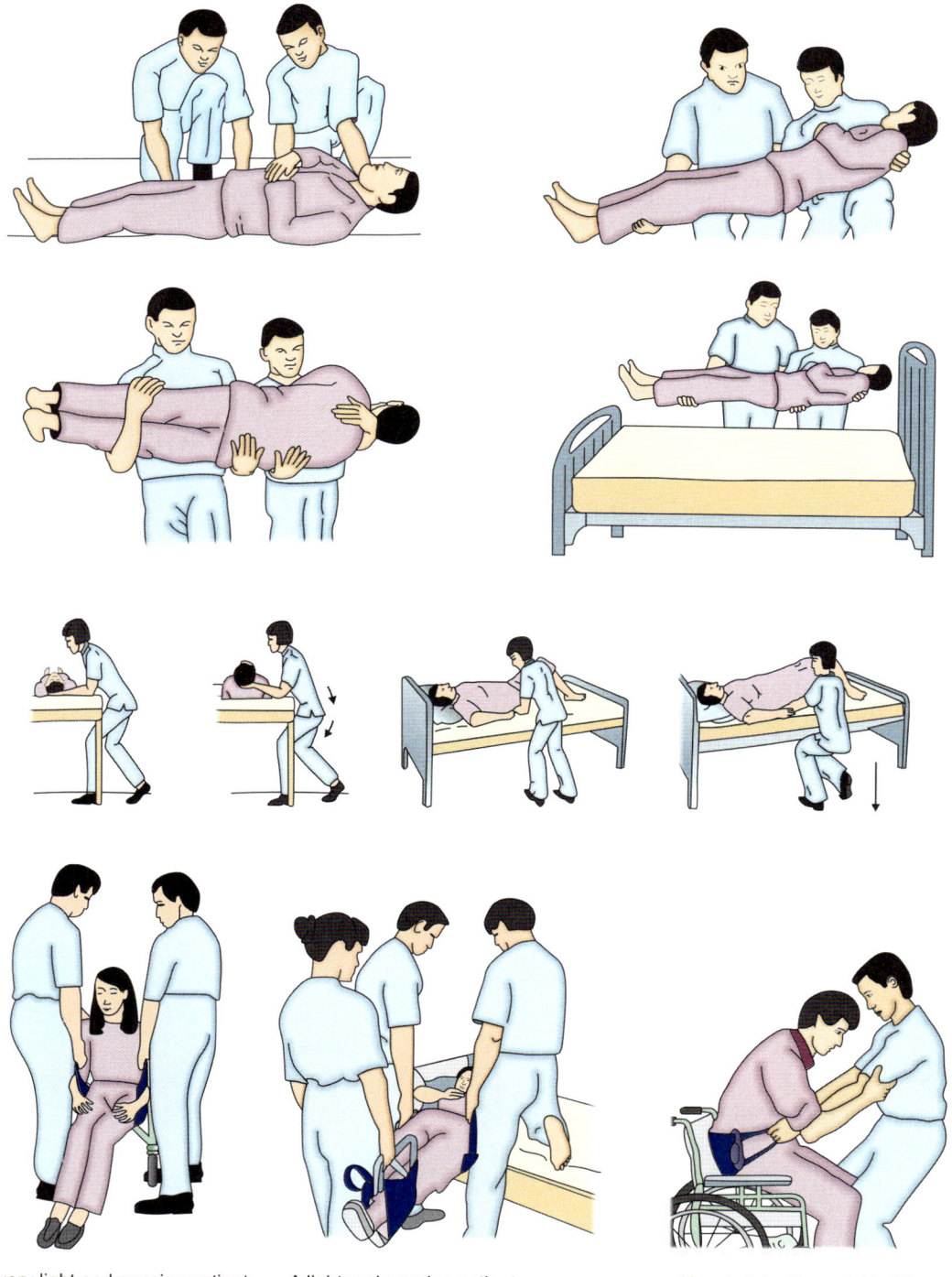

A very light and passive patient

A light and passive patient; helpers are using both a SST Sling and SSt Gumey

How to take the weight of the patient on to your body

Fig. 20.20: Nursing role in shifting client

Chapter 21

Endoscopy

Endoscopic Procedure

It is the use of flexible tube (the fiberoptic endoscope to visualize the GI tract and to perform certain diagnostic and therapeutic procedures. Images are produced through a video screen a tip of the endoscope moves in four directions, allowing for wide-angle visualization. The endoscope can be inserted through the rectum or mouth, depending on which portion of the GI tract is to be viewed. Endoscopes contain multipurpose channels that allow for air insufflation, irrigation, fluid aspiration, and the passage of special instrument. The instrument includes biopsy forceps, cytology brushes, needles, wire baskets, laser probes, and electrocautery snares. Its function other than visualization include biopsy or cytology of lesions, removal of foreign objects or polyps, control of internal bleeding, and opening of strictures.

Definition

The examination of a bodily orifice, canal or organ using an endoscope.

Purposes

1. To examine the organ
2. For therapeutic use
3. For diagnostic

Procedure Done in Hospital

1. EGD scopy (esophagogastroduodeno-scopy)
2. Colonoscopy
3. Sigmoidoscopy
4. Proctoscopy/proctosigmoidoscopy
5. Bronchoscopy

PREPARATION OF SCOPY ROOM

Preparation of Articles

1. Gastroscope (length 100 cm)—biopsy forceps, sclera needle
2. Banding set, peg set
3. Colonoscopy (length 160 cm)—biopsy forceps, polypsnar
4. Emergency resuscitation equipment and drugs
5. Suction apparatus, vital monitor, oxygen connection
6. Lubricant jelly, spray
7. Recording in the computer.

Esophagogastroduodenoscopy (EGD Scopy)

OGD scopy is a visualization of esophagus, stomach, duodenum by a flexible endoscope that permits biopsy cytology study pictures and video documentation.

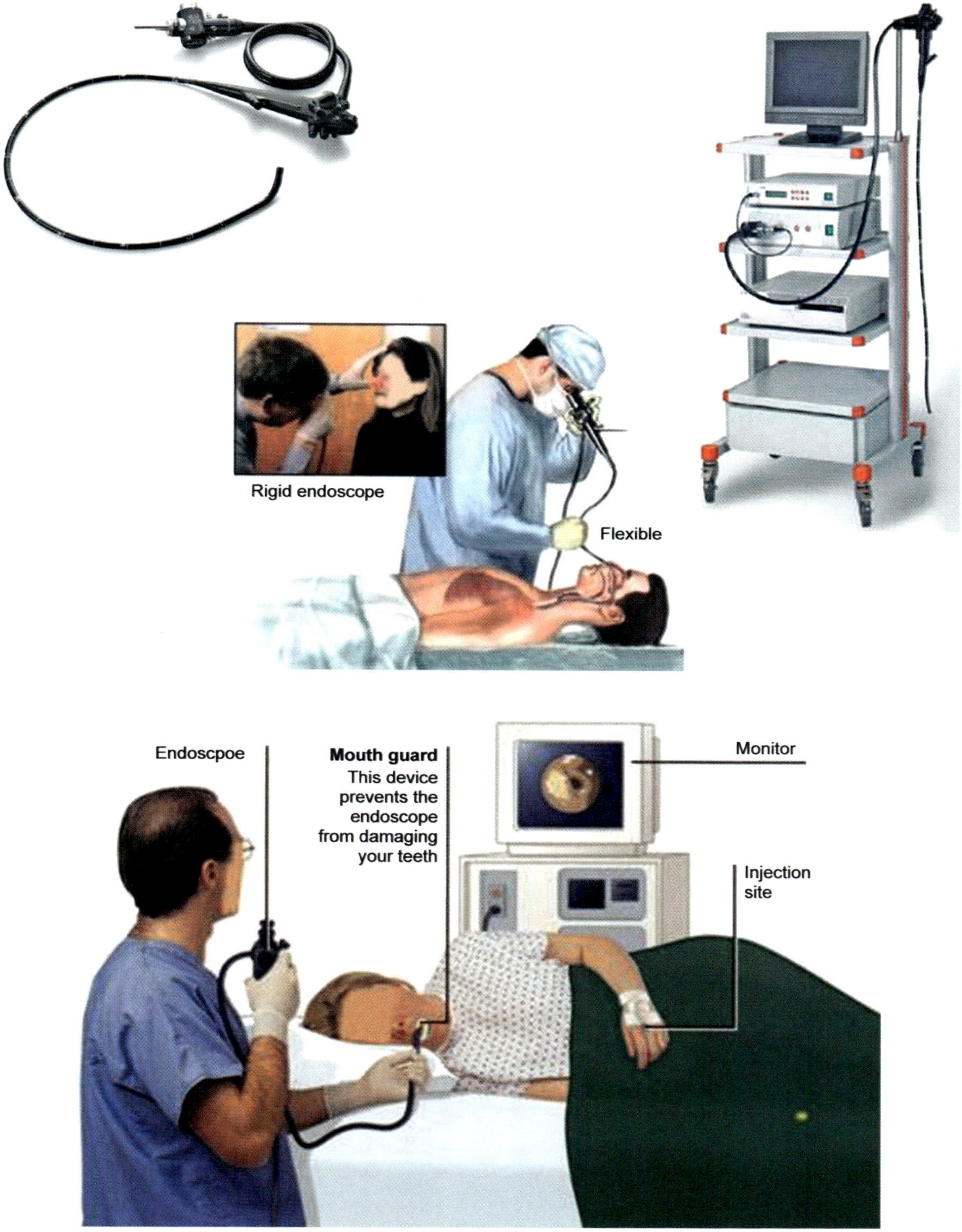

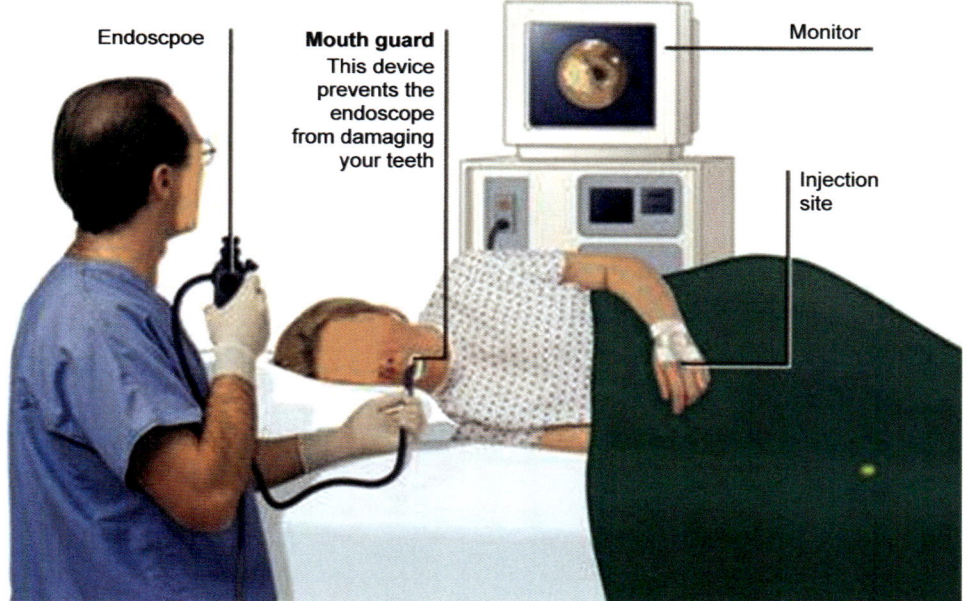

Rigid endoscope

Flexible

Endoscpoe

Mouth guard
This device
prevents the
endoscope
from damaging
your teeth

Monitor

Injection
site

Fig. 21.1: Visualization done by using endoscope

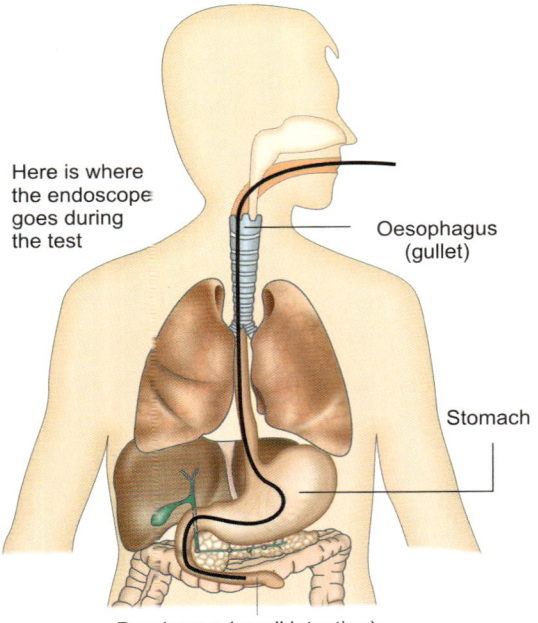

Here is where
the endoscope
goes during
the test

Oesophagus
(gullet)

Stomach

Duodenum (small intestine)

Fig. 21.2

Purposes

1. To perform biopsy/cytology study
2. To remove polyps and foreign bodies
3. To control bleeding (by sclerotherapy and banding)
4. To open stricture

Indication: Chronic bleeding, pernicious anemia, esophageal injury, mass in GI tract, stricture, dysphasia, substernal pain, ulcer, esophageal gastric varices, GERD

Pre-preparation of Client

1. Explain the procedure
2. Get informed consent
3. Keep client NBM for 8–12 hours
4. Assess the oral cavity and report any lesions or lose tooth, if dentures present remove it
5. Check for investigations, e.g. CBC, HIV, HBsAG, HCV (accordingly precautions can be taken)

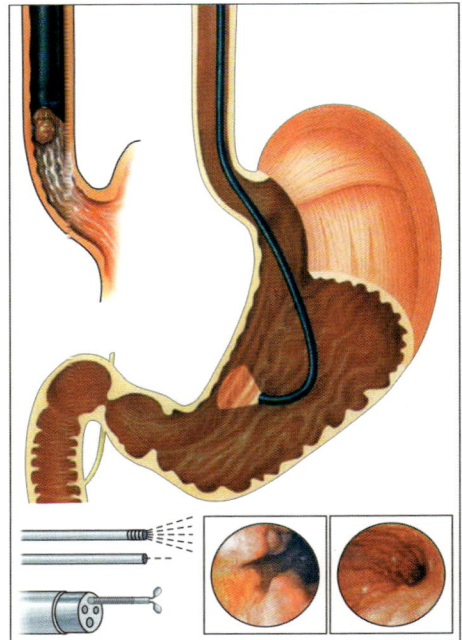

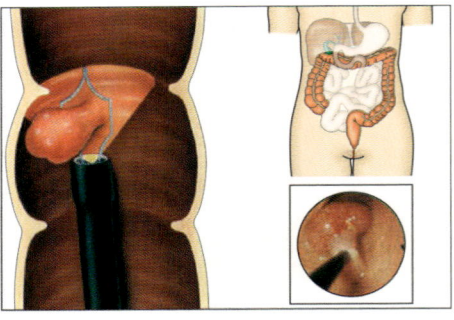

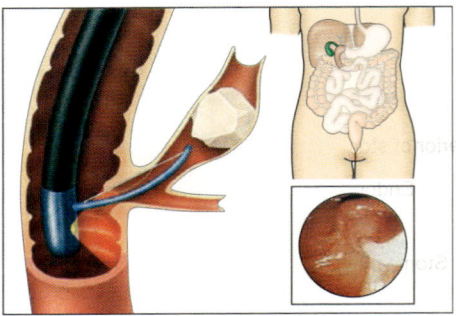

Fig. 21.3: Internal visuals of endoscopic procedure

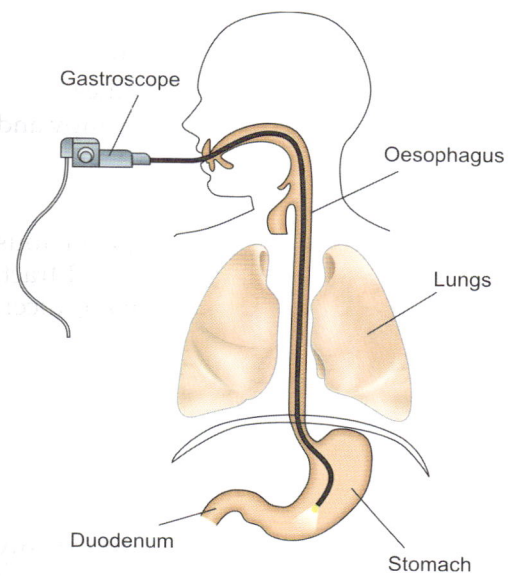

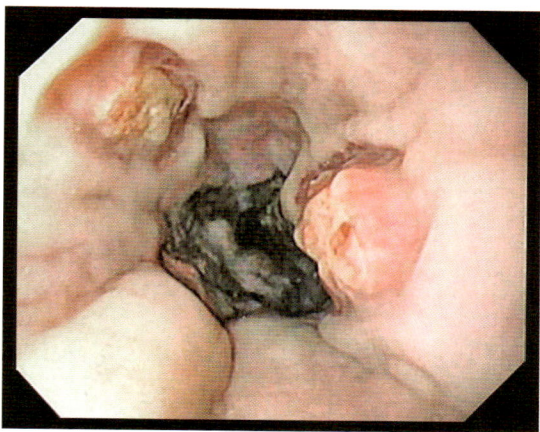

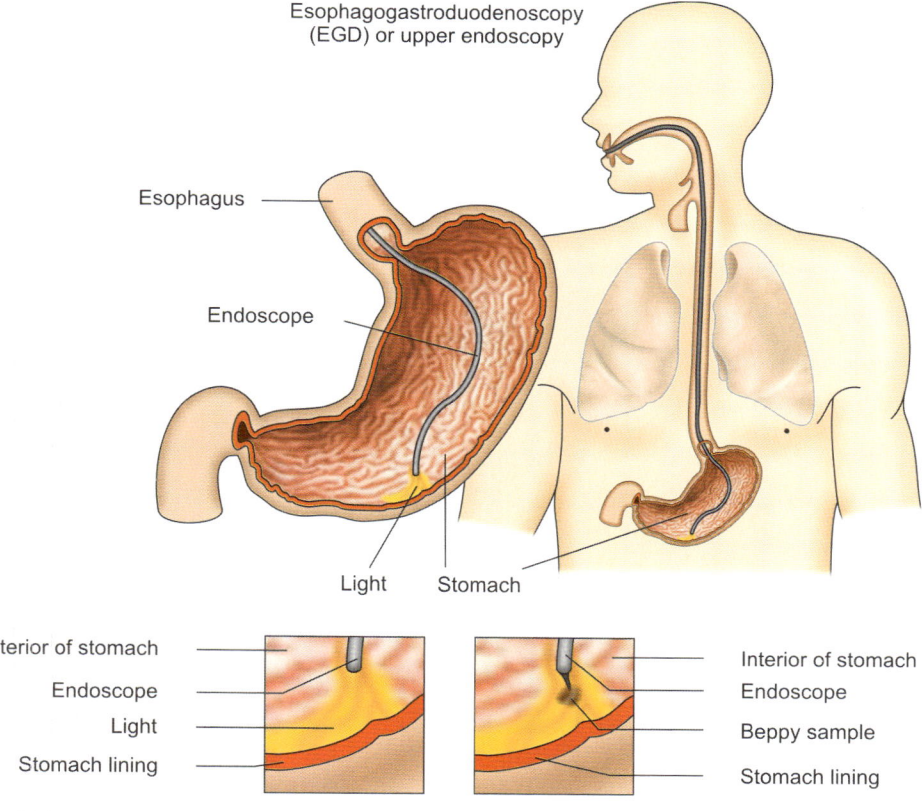

Fig. 21.4: Internal visuals of EGD scopy

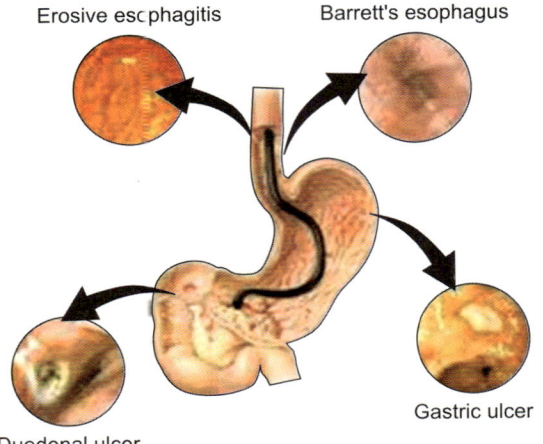

Erosive esophagitis

Barrett's esophagus

Duodenal ulcer

Gastric ulcer

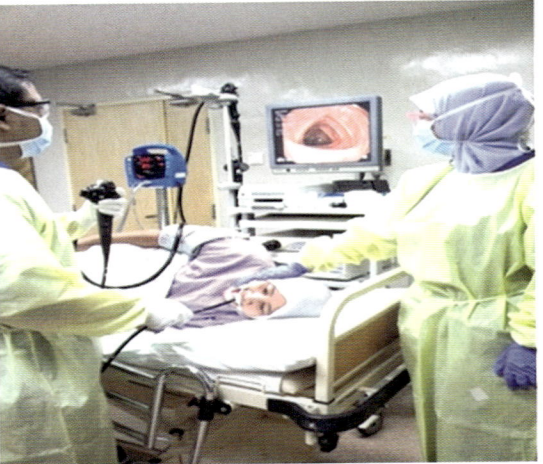

EGD scopy procedure

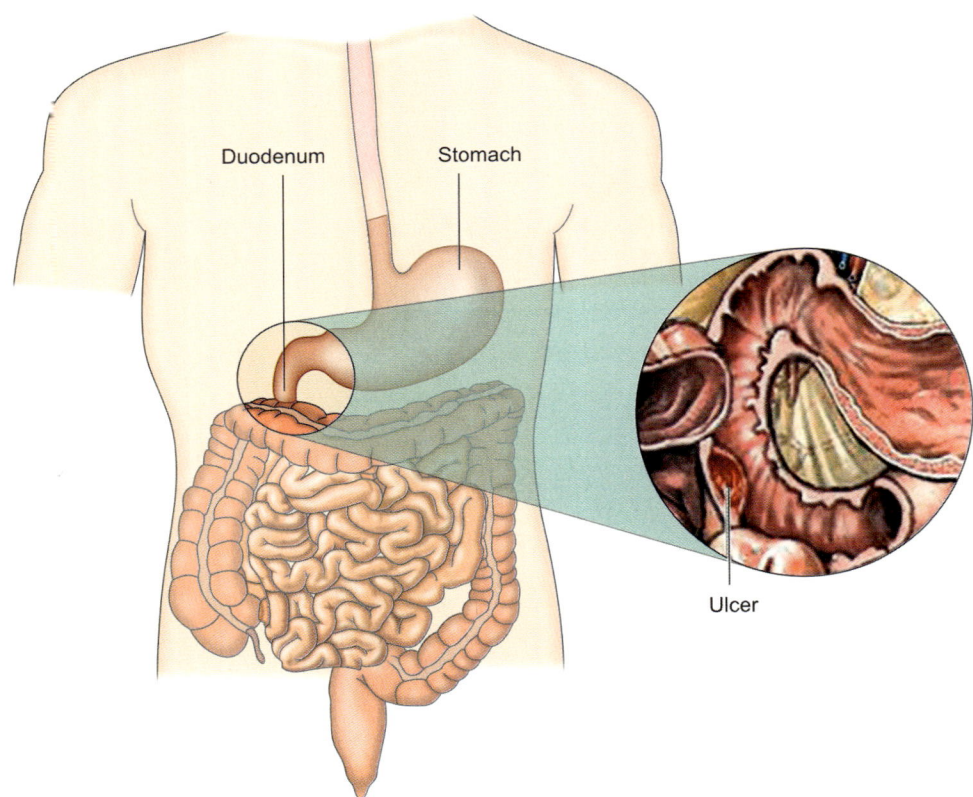

Duodenum

Stomach

Ulcer

Fig. 21.5: Anatomical location of ulcer

6. If client is on hypertensive drug can take the medication with sips of water.
7. Avoid diabetic medication and follow physicians order.

During Procedure

1. Enter in the computer record
2. Avoid speaking during procedure
3. Local anesthesia with spray done
4. Intravenous sedation given as per need
5. Client is given position left lateral
6. Endoscope is lubricated with water soluble jelly.
7. Mackintosh and towel is placed under the head of client.
8. Client is told to swallow the scope while it is inserted.
9. Suction any secretion note
10. Monitor vitals and oxygen saturation all through the procedure.

Post-procedure

1. Place the client is comfortable position
2. Client is kept under observation and monitoring for at least two hours.
3. Watch for any sigs of complications
4. Cleaning of scope such as suctioning, flushing, air chamber, etc.
5. If client is of HIV, HBSAG, HCV then the scope is placed in the cidex solution for 12 hours and discard the solution after use.
6. Details are enter into reporting
7. Document
8. Report is explained by doctor to the client
9. Handover of report file to client or his relatives.

Corresponding Procedure

1. Biopsy
2. Banding
3. Sclerotherapy
4. PEG tube insertion

Biopsy: Performed to get cytology report or to diagnose the clients condition.

Procedure

1. Explain procedure
2. Biopsy forceps sample is taken
3. Sample is preserved in normal saline and formalin
4. A sterile container is used
5. Label the sample
6. With biopsy letter from doctor sample is forwarded
7. Observe clients condition
8. Report in nurses record.

COLONOSCOPY

Colonoscopy is the visual examination of the lining of the rectum, colon and distal small bowel using a long flexible fiberoptic endoscope.

Purposes

1. To evaluate active or occult lower intestinal bleeding.
2. To identify abnormalities found on radiographic examination.
3. To diagnose suspected caecal or ascending colonic disease, anemia, cancer and inflammatory bowel disease.

Precaution: Fluid and electrolyte status of elderly clients and those with renal or cardiac disease to be considered during bowel preparation.

Oral Preparation

Explain the need of oral preparation.

Take peglec powder mixed with 1–2 liter water. Make a solution and finish the prepared solution within 1–2 hours. After that client will have the sensation to pass motion, client will have loose watery motion to clear bowel. Client may have 10–12 time motions. Do not throw the solution out by vomiting. After 4 hours client can have clear liquid like coconut water, lemon juice, fruit juice and energy drink.

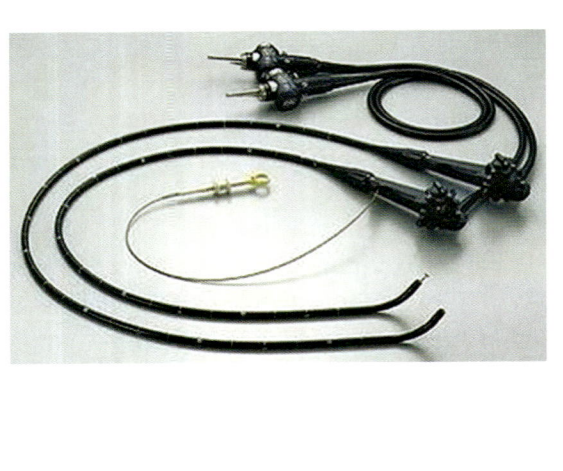

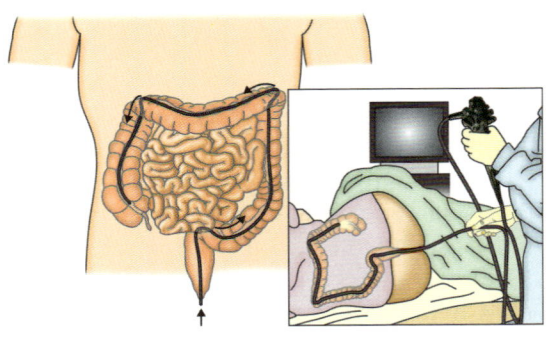

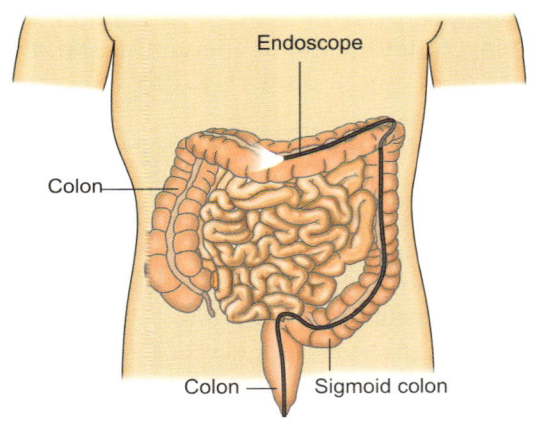

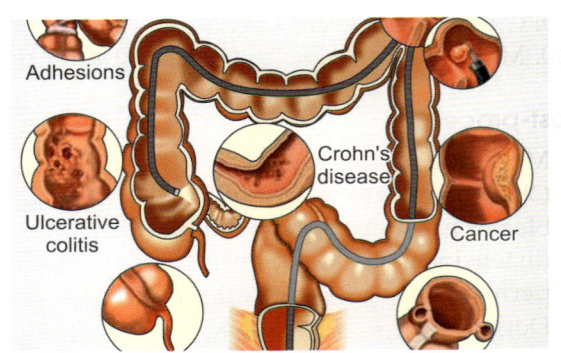

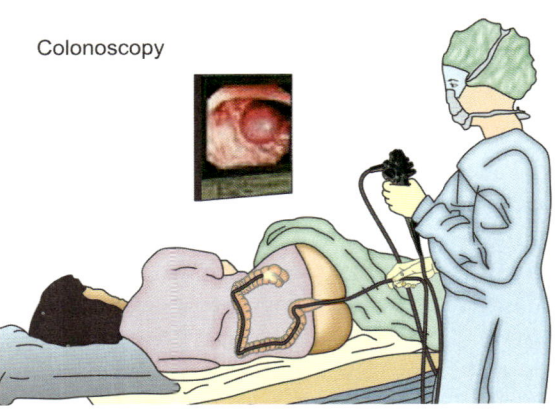

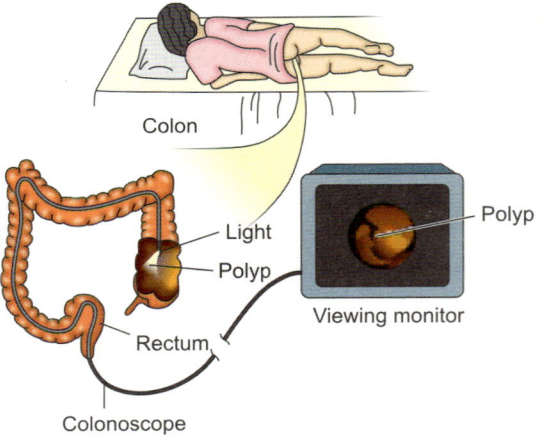

Fig. 21.6: Colonoscopy procedure and its visuals in different angles

Keep client 12 hours NBM

IV cannulation done if mild sedation ordered.

During Procedure

1. Explain the procedure
2. Get informed consent
3. Maintain the privacy of client
4. Monitor vitals and levels of consciousness
5. If ordered give IV medication (sedation)
6. Instruct client to take deep slow breath during the scope being inserted.
7. Apply pressure to areas of abdomen as directed by doctor as the scope passes through the spleen flexure, caecum.
8. Monitor abdominal distension, pain, tolerance
9. Clean genital area
10. Make documentation.

Post-procedure

1. Monitor and document vitals for one hour
2. Observe signs of complication like rectal bleeding, vomiting, severe abdominal pain, distension, rigidity which are indication of perforation.
3. Document response of procedure of client
4. Client may feel distended due to gas introduced to visualize organs.

SIGMOIDOSCOPY

Sigmoidoscopy visualization of rectum to internal bowel of sigmoid region in condition to see rectal mass, ulcer, bleeding piles.

Procedure

1. Keep the client for 12 hours
2. Give simple enema before 2 hours of scopy
3. Document procedure

Sclera therapy: Injection slerosing agent introduced through a flexible endoscope into the bleeding esophageal varices to promote thrombosis.

Purposes

1. To treat client with actually bleeding
2. To treat client with portal hypertension
3. To treat client with hemorrhoids

Articles

1. Gastroscope with large biopsy channel
2. Injection adrenaline
3. Injector needle
4. Emergency resuscitation equipment
5. Medications/drugs

Procedure

1. Explain procedure
2. Get informed consent
3. Provide instruction about pre-procedure on the method of procedure.
4. Identify any contraindication, review physicians orders for pre-procedure medication.
5. Instruct the client to remain NBM in the night before the procedure if sclerotherapy (for hemorrhoids) done on upper gastrointestinal tract.
6. Ensure that bowel preparation
7. Place the client in left lateral position
8. Place mouth gauge if upper GI tract method.
9. Assist the doctor to injector through the scope
10. Ensure clients comfort and monitor vitals, complications before sifting the client to day care unit.
11. Record the procedure and handover reports to clients relatives.
12. Transfer client to day care unit.

PERCUTANEOUS ENDOSCOPIC GASTROTOMY PEG TUBE

This tube inserted by using fiberoptic endoscope with peg tube to feed directly through the stomach in several cases like cancer esophagus, paralysis, cancer trachea, bedridden client.

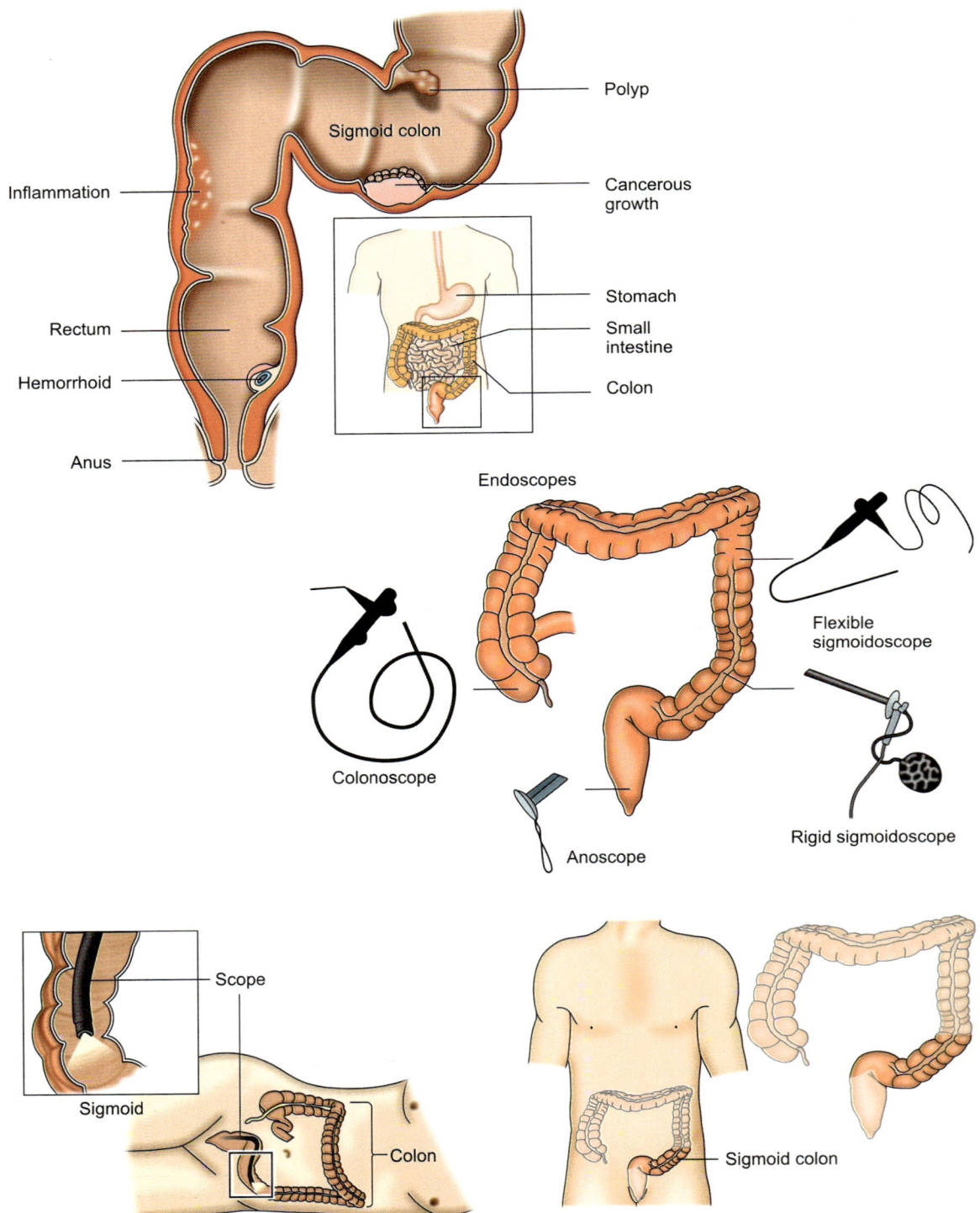

Fig. 21.7: Anatomical site of sigmoidoscopy

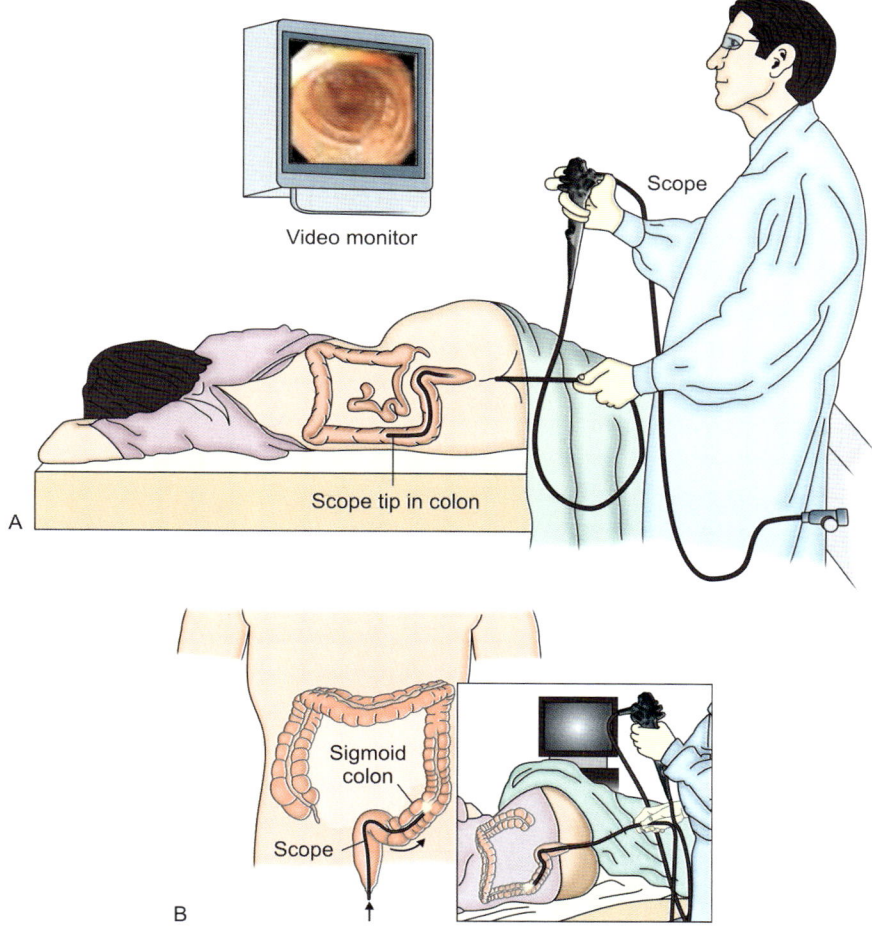

Fig. 21.8A and B: Sigmoidoscopy

Purposes

1. To give supplementary diet to the client
2. To maintain balance diet

Articles

1. Monitor, oxygen source, emergency drug
2. Endoscope, lubricant jelly spray
3. Peg set with peg tube sterile articles
4. Sterile kidney tray, gown, mask, cap, gloves

Procedure

1. Explain the procedure
2. Get informed consent
3. Give premedication as order by doctor
4. Prepare trolley and maintain sterility of the articles
5. Give position to client
6. Assist the doctor while he places peg tube
7. Clamp the tube, do the dressing after procedure
8. Monitor the vitals and any complications during procedure
9. Get the permission for anesthetic before shifting client
10. Observe client for secretion, discomfort, pain
11. Give IV fluids as ordered

12. Client is kept NBM till physicians order
13. Document in nurses notes
14. Transfer/shift the client to the ward
15. During handover explain about care of the peg tube, feeding, etc.

PROCTOSCOPY

Proctoscopy is an endoscopic direct visual examination of the lining of rectum and anal canal using a rigid lighted proctoscopy.

Purposes

1. To asses and evaluate for rectal bleeding
2. Hemorrhoids
3. Polyps cysts
4. Blood or mucus in the stool
5. Unexplained anemia
6. Chronic constipation
7. Rectal/anal ulceration
8. Condition of anus/rectum before surgery

Contraindication

1. Severe necrotizing enterocolitis
2. Toxic megacolon
3. Painful anal lesions
4. Severe cardiac dysrhythmias

Articles

1. Protoscope
2. Clean gloves
3. 1–2% lidocaine (xylocaine)
4. Specimen container with 10% formalin
5. Cytology slides and jar with 95% ethyl alcohol
6. Sterile swabs with culture tubes
7. Lubricant
8. Cotton swabs
9. Emesis basin
10. Biopsy forceps
11. Receptacle

Procedure

Pre-procedure

1. Explain procedure to patient benefits of test and risk involved

2. Obtain informed consent
3. Inform client for restricted diet such as clear liquids in the evening before the test
4. Laxative or enema given before night examination. Morning laxative suppository may be administered
5. Wash hands
6. Assemble articles
7. Don hospital gown
8. Provide privacy

During Procedure

1. Position client in knee chest. Weak and ill client give sims position
2. Assist assistance in helping client maintain position
3. Don gloves
4. Continue instructing client during progress of procedure
5. Apply lubricant to gloved finger
6. Insert lubricant finger in rectum to check the possible obstruction prior to insertion of protoscope.
7. Lubricate end of the protoscope
8. Physician gently inserts endoscope into anal canal as required.
9. If cramping occurs the client may require more medication or temporary pause in the forward movement of the scope.
10. Advice client to breath through mouth when scope insertion
11. Slowly remove endoscope at complexion of examination
12. Place endoscope in appropriate container with cleaning
13. Remove soiled gloves and place in appropriate receptacle

After Procedure

1. Wash hands
2. Send specimen to lab immediately
3. Ask client to lie flat position for 10 to 15 minutes.
4. Monitor for signs of fatigue, abdominal pain or distension, fever, hypertension or rectal bleeding.

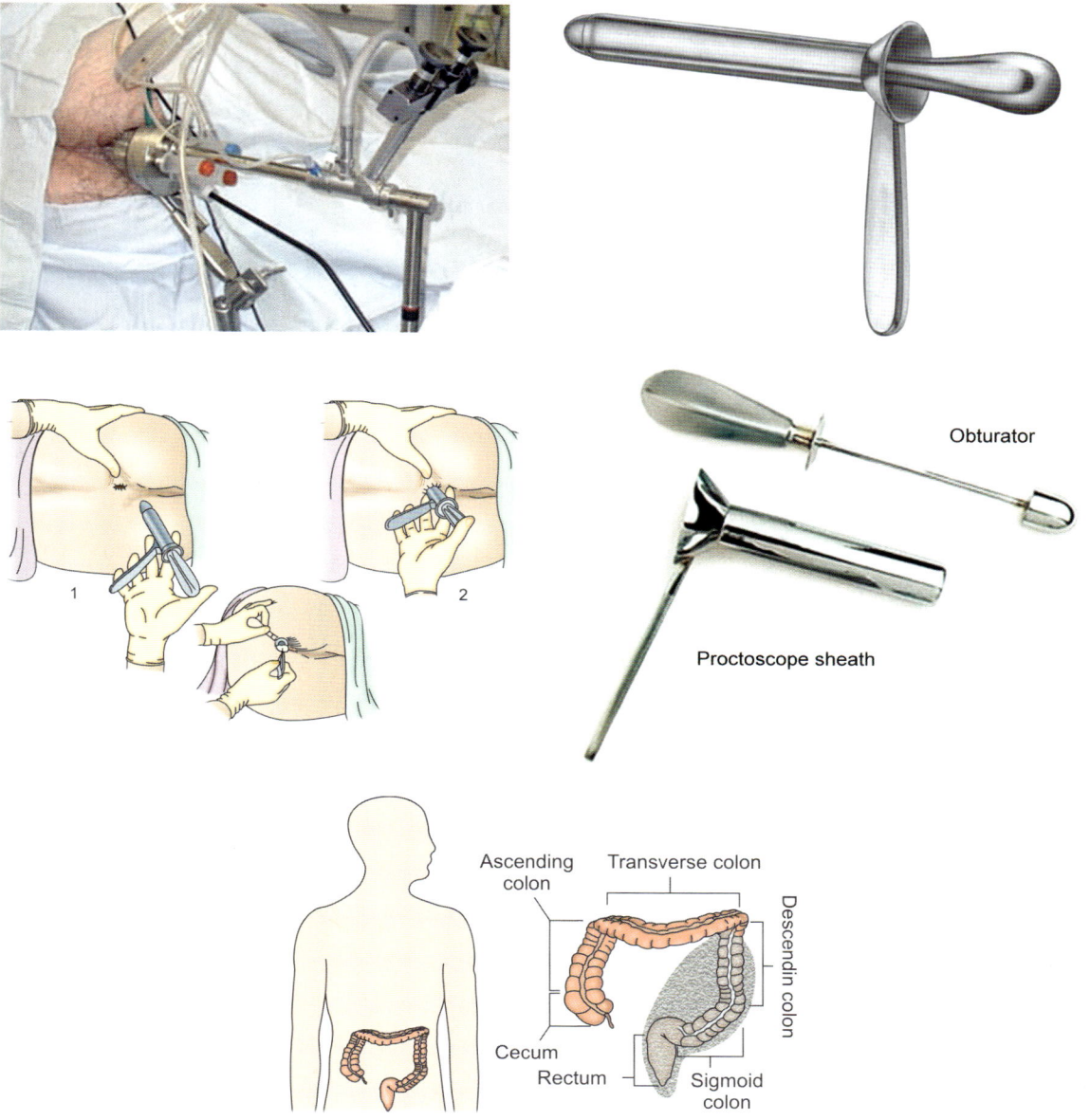

Fig. 21.9: Proctoscopy instrument insertion site

5. Observe for possible complications such as rectal perforation, persistent abdominal discomfort, rectal bleeding, fever.
6. Special consideration no enema or barium studies should be performed for one week following rectal biopsy as there is increased risk of perforation.

BRONCHOSCOPY

Assisting with direct inspection and examination of the larynx, trachea and bronchi through either or flexible fiberoptic bronchoscope or a rigid bronchoscope (the fiberoptic scope allows for less discomfort and better visualization of smaller airways).

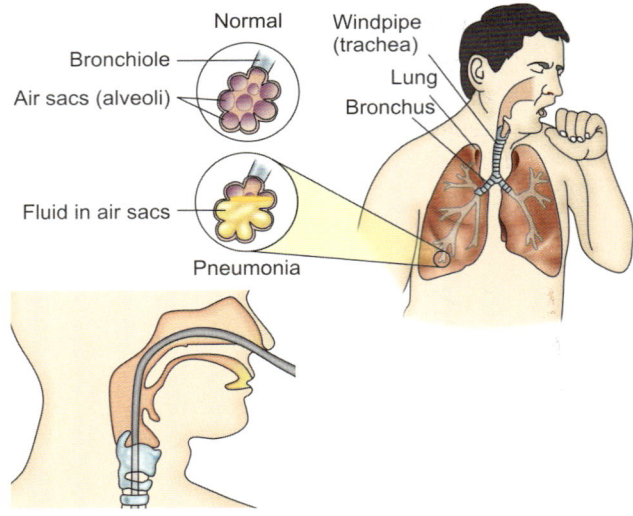

Normal
Bronchiole
Air sacs (alveoli)
Windpipe (trachea)
Lung
Bronchus
Fluid in air sacs
Pneumonia

A bronchoscope is used to view the airways and check for any abnormalities

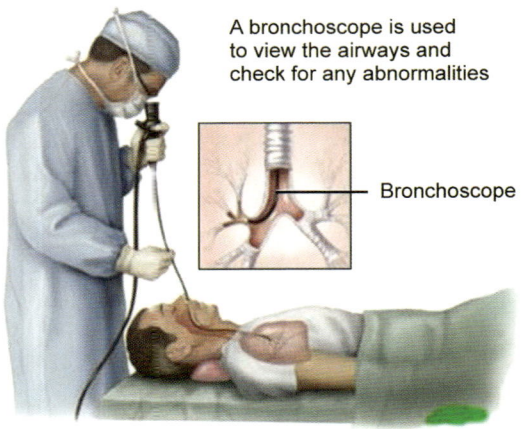

Bronchoscope

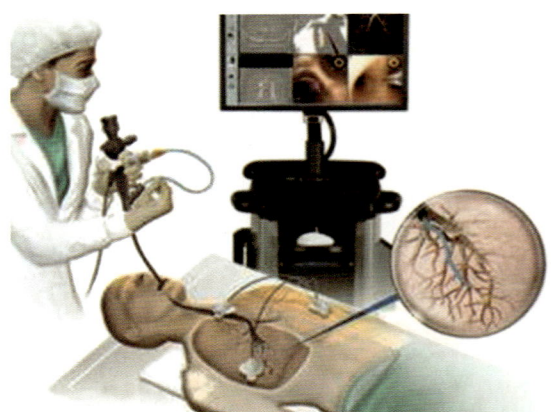

Camera
Fiberoptic bronchoscope
Bronchi Light Trachea

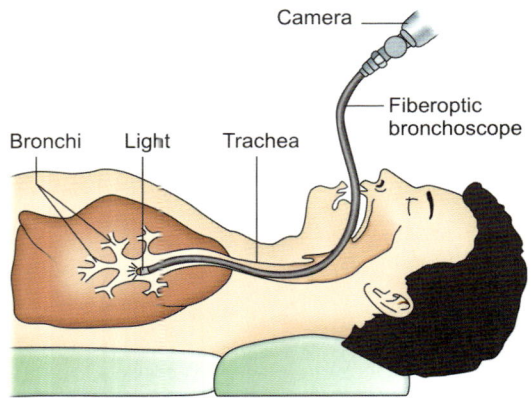

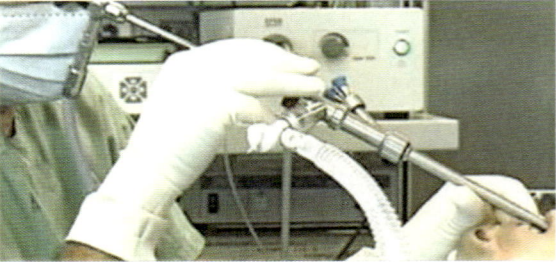

Fig. 21.10: Visualization through bronchoscope instrument

Diagnostic Purpose

1. For examination of tissue
2. For further evaluation of a tumor for potential surgical resection
3. To collect tissue specimen for diagnosis
4. Evaluate bleeding sites

Therapeutic Purpose

1. To remove foreign bodies
2. To remove thick, viscous secretions
3. To treat postoperative
4. To remove and destroy lesions

Procedure

Pre-procedure

1. Explain the procedure to obtain cooperation and provide reassurance
2. Obtain informed consent
3. Remove dentures, contact lens and other prosthesis before procedure to prevent interference with the procedure.
4. Instruct client to be on NPO for 6–12 hours before procedure to reduce the risk of aspiration during procedure.
5. Administer pre-medications as per physician's instruction. It inhibits vagal stimulation.
6. Spray topical anesthetic lignocain as the pharynx to suppress cough reflex and minimize discomfort.
7. Administer sedatives intravenously as prescribed.
8. Instruct client to lie supine with head hyper extended.
9. Monitor vital signs, oz saturation, cardiac rhythm and reassure client during the procedure.

Post-procedure Care

1. Monitor vital signs
2. Observe the client for signs of respiratory changes
3. Inspect expectorated secretions for hemoptysis
4. Keep client on NPO until gag reflex returns
5. Give ice chips and small sips of water when client regains swallowing reflex.
6. Monitor lung sounds for 24 hours
7. Instruct the client and family to report any shortness of breath or bleeding immediately.

Complications

1. Pneumothorax
2. Dysrhythmias
3. Bronchospasm
4. Infection
5. Aspiration
6. Perforation

Chapter 22

Anesthesia

Anesthesia can be classified into:
1. General anesthesia
2. Regional/local anesthesia
3. Spinal anesthesia (subarachnoid block: SAB)
4. Topical (surface) anesthesia
5. A nerve block
6. An intravenous block (Bier block)
7. Epidural anesthesia

General anesthesia is loss of all sensation and consciousness. Under this anesthesia, protective reflexes such as cough and gag reflexes are lost. GA are usually administered by intravenous infusion or by inhalation of gases through a mask or through an endotracheal tube inserted into the trachea.

   i. *Nitrous oxide* is stored in cylinders in a liquid form, under pressure, often referred to as gases. Nitrous oxide is a weak anesthetic agent of high concentration.

   ii. *Ether,* a volatile liquid which is rarely used now has a wide margin of safety. Although prolonged inhalation can cause postoperative vomiting and deep. Although prolonged inhalation can cause postoperative vomiting and depression, it has an unpleasant, irritant smell, it is inflammable and explosive when mixed with oxygen.

   iii. *Halothane (fluothane),* a volatile liquid which is neither flammable nor expulsive. Its characteristic is no irritation to respiratory tract.

   iv. **Isoflurane (aerrane forane),** this is an isomer of influrance and although able to produce a more rapid induction than halothane, is more irritant which reduces its usefulness

   v. **Sevoflurane**—non-flammable and non-explosive which are in form of inhalation types of anesthesia.

Regional/local anesthesia is the temporary interruption of the transmission of nerve impulses to and from a specific area or region of the body but remains conscious. Several techniques are used.

Local anesthesia (infiltration) is injected into a specific area and is used for minor surgical procedure such as surgery of small wound or performing a biopsy. Lidocaine or tetracaine 0.1% may be used.

A nerve block is a technique in which the anesthetic agent is injected into and around the nerve or small nerve group that supplies sensation to a small area of the body. Major blocks involves multiple nerves or a plexus, e.g. the volve a single nerve, a facial nerve.

An intravenous block (Bier block) is used more often for procedures involving the arm,

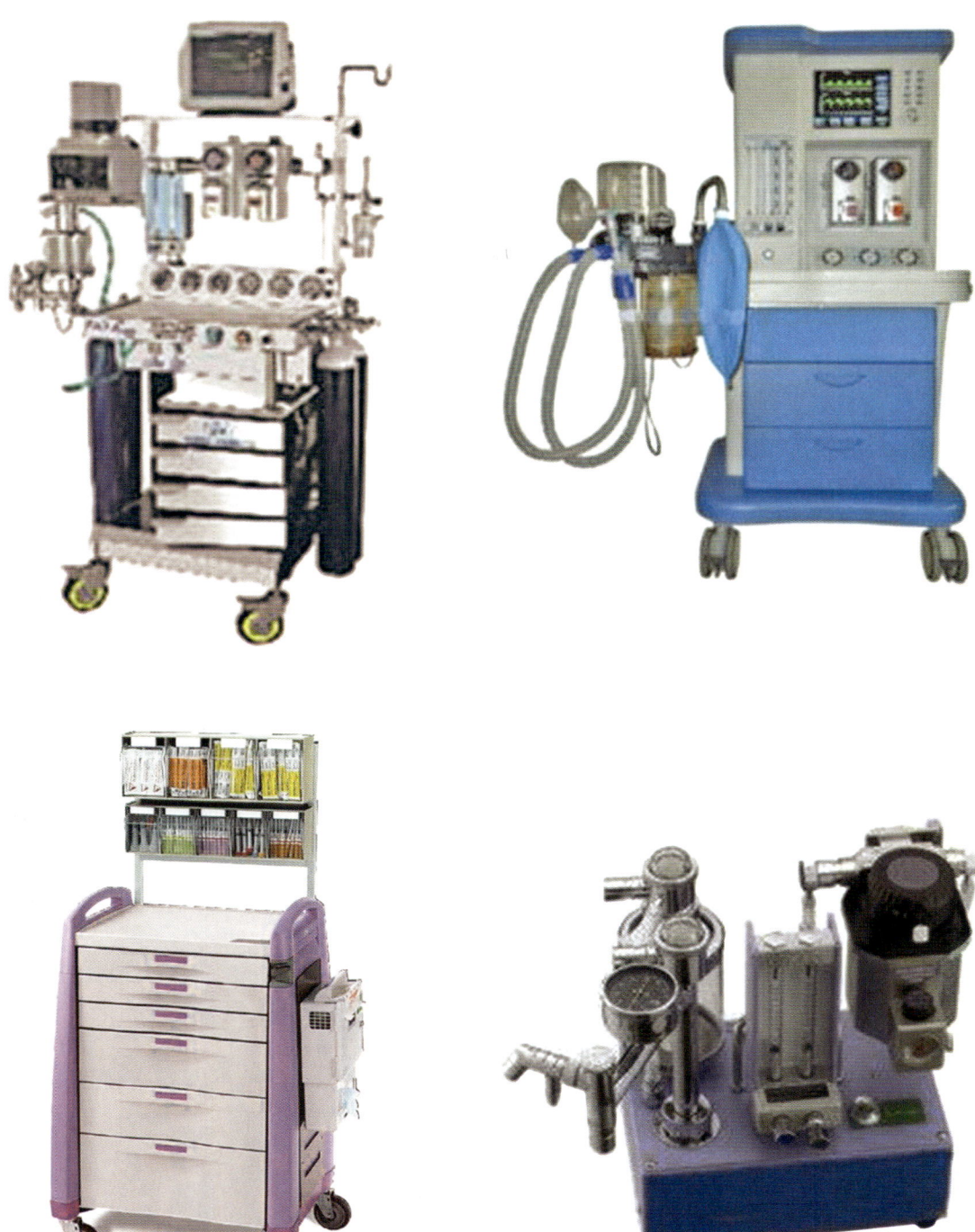

Fig. 22.1: Anesthesia trolly in OT room—different models in use

wrist, and hand. An occlusion tourniquet is applied to the extremity to prevent infiltration and absorption of the injected intravenous agent beyond the involved extremity

Spinal anesthesia is also referred to as subarachnoid block (SAB). It requires a lumbar puncture through one of the interspaces between lumbar disc 2 (L2) and the sacrum (S1). An anesthetic agent is injected into a subachnoid space surrounding the spinal cord. Spinal anesthesia is often categorized as a low, mid, or high spinal. Low spinals are used for surgeries involving the perineal or rectal areas. Mid spinals (below levels of umbilicaus-T10) can be used for hernia repairs or appendectomies, and high spinals (reaching the nipple line-T4) can be used for surgeries such as cesarean sections.

Epidural (peridural) anesthesia is an injection of an anesthetic agent into the epidural space, the area inside the spinal column but outside the dura mater.

Anesthesia Apparatus

1. Anesthetic gas cylinders—anesthetic gas cylinders are colored in accordance with a British standards institute code. Oxygen cylinders are painted black with a white top and oxygen printed in black.
2. Nitrous oxide is blue with NZO printed in black
3. Cyclopropane is orange with C3H6 printed in black
4. Carbon dioxide is painted grey with Coz also in black.

General anesthesia does not require the anesthetic machine tested daily as basic equipment. Anesthesia machines may differ in appearance, size, and degree of sophistication but generally speaking, they consist of suction for:
   i. Ventilation
   ii. Accessories
   iii. Storage space
   iv. Worktop

It is imperative that essential medical pipeline gas supply.

Articles

1. The respirator bag valve mask
2. Anesthesia machine
3. Oxygen mask
4. Laryngoscope
5. Tracheotomy tube
6. Tuohy needle
7. Flexible endoscope
8. Syringe
9. Spinal needles
10. Non-kink catheter mount.

Doctor's use Drug

1. Injection fulsed
2. Injection propofol
3. Injection pento
4. Injection ketamine
5. Injection scolin
6. Injection Tracrium
7. Injection lox heavy
8. Injection anawin heavy

Emergency Drug Trolley

1. Injection fortwin and injection atropine
2. Injection sodiumbicarbonate
3. Injection Kcl
4. Injection aminophylline
5. Injection efcorlin
6. Injection deriphylline
7. Injection lasix
8. Injection adrenaline
9. Injection emeset
10. Injection pause
11. Injection D 25%
12. Injection calcium gluconate
13. Injection dopamine
14. Injection NTG
15. Injection dexamethasone

Three trays of anesthetic drugs to be always keep ready in the fridge.

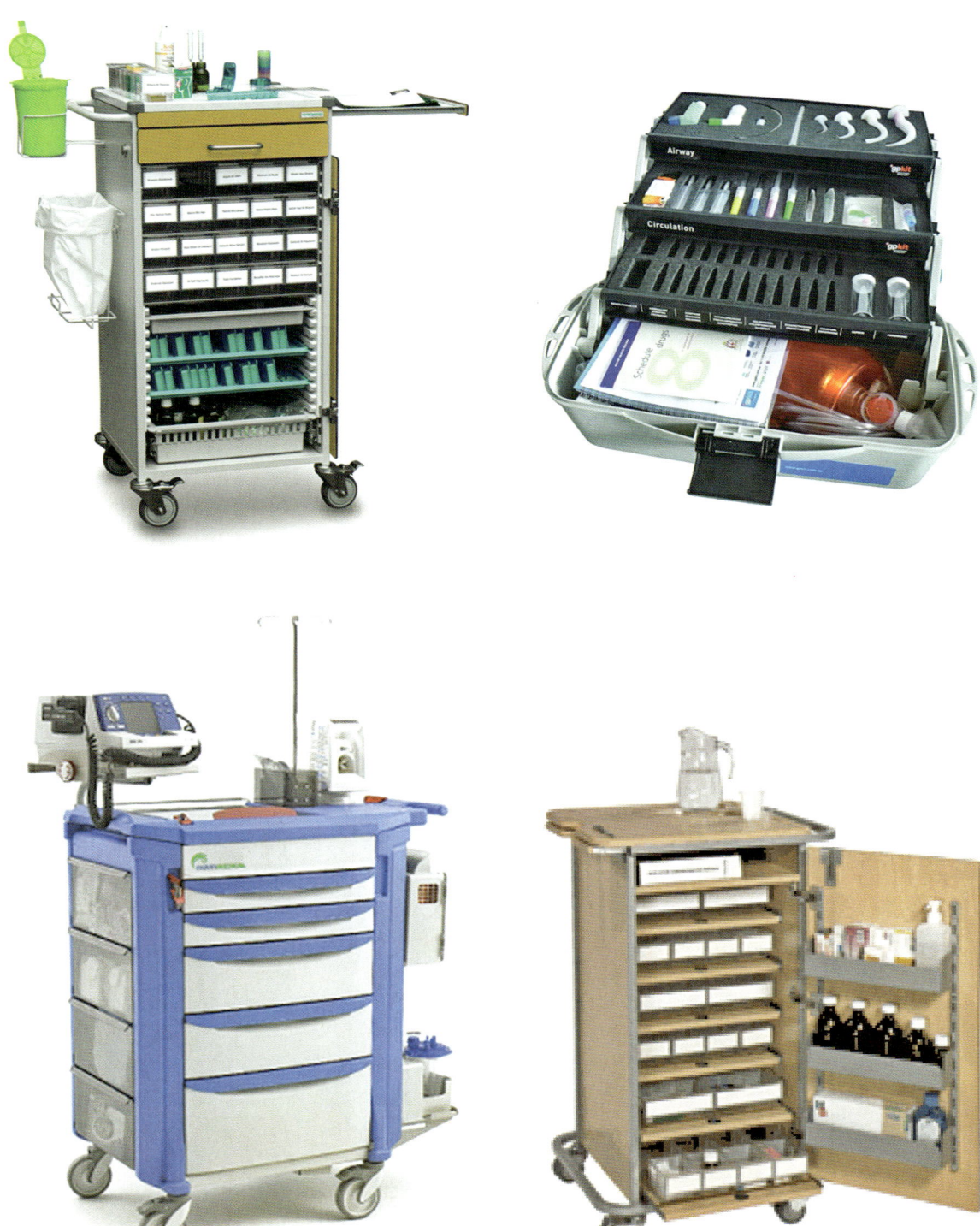

Fig. 22.2: Emergency drugs trolly

After using drug before keeping the tray in place it should be check and replace the injection

Every evening on while closing the OT the anesthetic tray should be checked again

Pre-anesthetic care

During/intra-anesthetic care

Post-anesthetic are should be added

No need of explaining equipment used in anesthesia.

Nurses role in care of preoperative client

Classification of surgery.

Chapter 23

Thoracentesis

Definition

Thoracentesis is insertion of a needle into the pleural space to remove accumulated fluid and air using aseptic technique or thoracentesis is the aspiration of pleural fluid or air for diagnostic or therapeutic purpose by a doctor with the assistance of a nurse.

Purposes

1. To remove air and fluid from pleural cavity
2. To decrease pressure on the lung tissue
3. To aspirate pleural fluid for diagnostic studies.
4. To instill medication into the pleural space
5. To installation of medication into pleural space.

Articles

Pleural Aspiration Set

a. Sponge holding forceps
b. 5 ml syringe with needle
c. 20 ml syringe with liver lock
d. Aspiration needle No. 264
e. Two small bowels
f. Dissecting forceps
g. Artery forceps
h. Specimen bottles and slides
i. Gown, mask and gloves
j. Sterile dressing towel
k. Cotton swabs, gauze pieces and pads
l. Scalpel blade

Clean Tray

1. Mackintosh and towel
2. Kidney tray and paper bag
3. Spirit, povidone iodine
4. Lignocain 2%
5. Adhesive plaster and scissors
6. Tincture Benzoin

Other Articles

1. Cardiac table or back rest, as needed
2. Pillow

Procedure

Pre-procedure

1. Identify client and explain procedure to client and his relatives
2. Explain that during procedure client may experience a sensation of deep pressure when fluid is aspirated
3. Review the chest X-ray
4. Obtain an informed consent from client
5. Instruct clients that he should not move during procedure as it can cause injury to vital organs or blood vessels
6. Position client comfortably. An upright position facilitated localization of fluid at the bas of the chest. Sitting on the edge of the bed with the feet supported arms and head on pillow over the cardiac table.
7. Expose the client for physician to determine the site of aspiration by

Thoracentesis

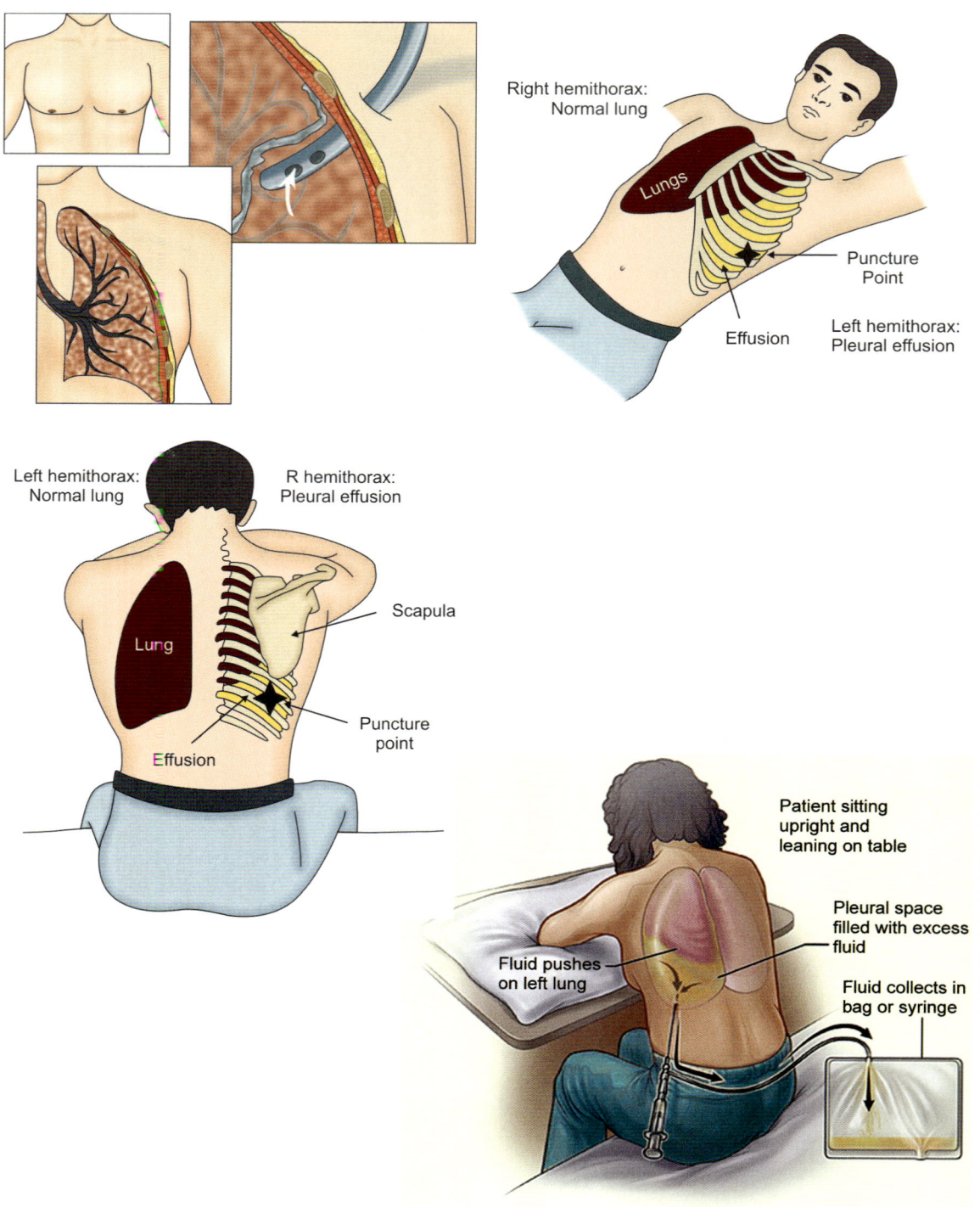

Fig. 23.1: Site of thoracentesis procedure and its position

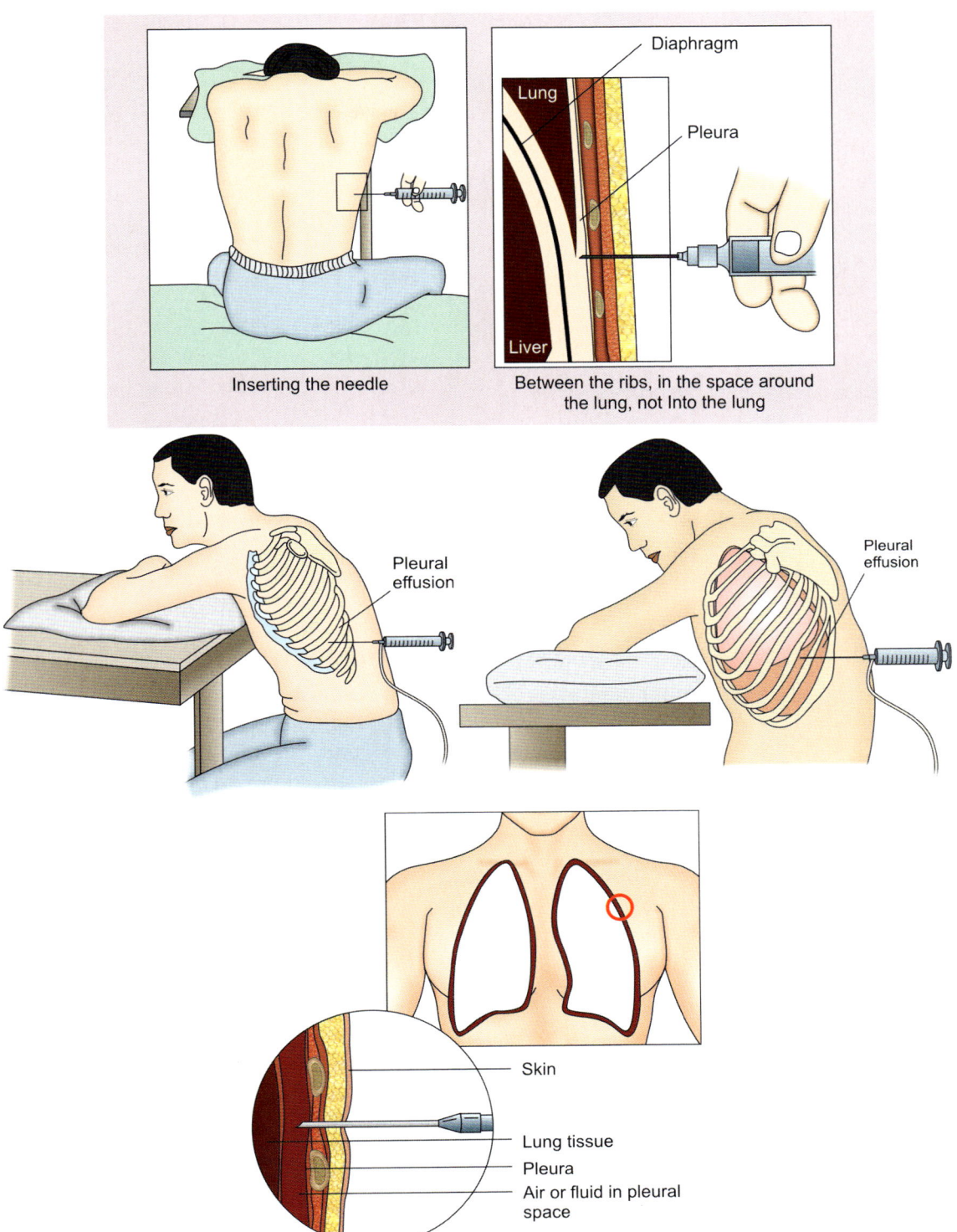

Fig. 23.2: Site of puncture of thoracentesis procedure

visualizing chest X-ray and performing chest percussion.

8. If air to be removed the site is usually in 2nd and 3rd intercostals space.
9. If fluid is removed the site is usually 8th and 9th intercostals space.
10. Clean the site with antiseptic solution and assist the physician in administering local anesthesia.
11. The physician introduces the thoracentesis needle. Advice client to hold his breath when needle is inserted. As respiratory movement can cause risk of puncture to vital organs.
12. When needle is in pleural space, physician aspirates pleural fluid with syringe. Assist in collecting specimen in sterile containers.
13. A 20 ml syringe with a 3 way adapter is attached to needle. 3 way adapter helps to prevent air entering the pleural cavity when large volumes of fluid is removed.
14. Monitor vital sings.

During Procedure

Observe a strict aseptic technique during the procedure.

After Procedure

1. Send labeled specimen to lab

2. Instruct client to do deep breathing and coughing exercise. Demonstrate and teach these exercises to client
3. Have a post chest X-ray if indicated
4. Around 1000 to 1200 ml of fluid is removed and 30 to 60 ml of fluid is send for diagnostic purpose.
5. After needle is withdrawn, apply tincture Benzoin seal and pressure dressing over the site.
6. Monitor vitals every 30 minutes. Complication may occur because of accidental puncture of vital organs of blood vessels.
7. Closely watch the client after the procedure for 2 to 3 hours.
8. Record the procedure with total amount of fluid withdrawn color, nature and signs of complications.
9. Wash hands and articles used for procedure in cold water and then in warm soapy water. Rinse, dry and send for autoclaving, wear gloves while washing.

Complications

1. Pneumothorax
2. Subcutaneous emphysema
3. Phylogenic infection
4. Pulmonary edema
5. Cardiac distress

Chapter 24

Performing Neonatal Resuscitation and Chest Compression

Definition

Measures taken to review newborns who have difficulty in establishing respiration at birth and includes suctioning, positive pressure ventilation, external cardiac massage, intubation and medications as necessitated by the neonates condition at one minute after birth.

Purposes

1. To establish and maintain a clear airway
2. To ensure effective circulation
3. To correct any acidosis present
4. To prevent hypothermia, hypoglycemia and hemorrhage.

ARTICLES

Suctioning Articles

1. Bulb syringe
2. De lee mucous trap with no. 10 Fr. catheter or mechanical suction
3. Suction catheters no. 6, 8, 10
4. Feeding tube no. Fr. and 20 ml syringe

Bag and Mask Articles

1. Infant resuscitation bag with pressure release valve or pressure gauge with reservoir, capable of delivering 90–100% oxygen.
2. Face masks with cushioned rims (newborn and premature sizes)
3. Oral airways (newborn and premature sizes)
4. Oxygen with flow meter and tubing.

Intubation Articles

1. Laryngoscope with straight blades No. "0" (premature), No. "1" (newborn)
2. Extra bulbs and batteries for laryngoscope
3. Endotracheal tubes. Sizes—2.5, 3.0. 3.5 and 4.0 mm internal diameter
4. Stylet
5. Scissors

Medications

1. Epinephrine 1:10,000 ampoules (1 ml ampoule of 1:1,000 available in India)
2. Nalaxone hydrochloride (neonatal narcan 0.02 mg/ml)
3. Volume expander—5% albumin solution, normal saline, ringers lactate
4. Sodium bicarbonate 4.2% (1 mEq/2 ml) 7.5% strength available in India is approximately 0.9 mEq/ml.
5. Dextrose 10% concentration 250 ml
6. Sterile water 30 ml
7. Normal saline 30 ml

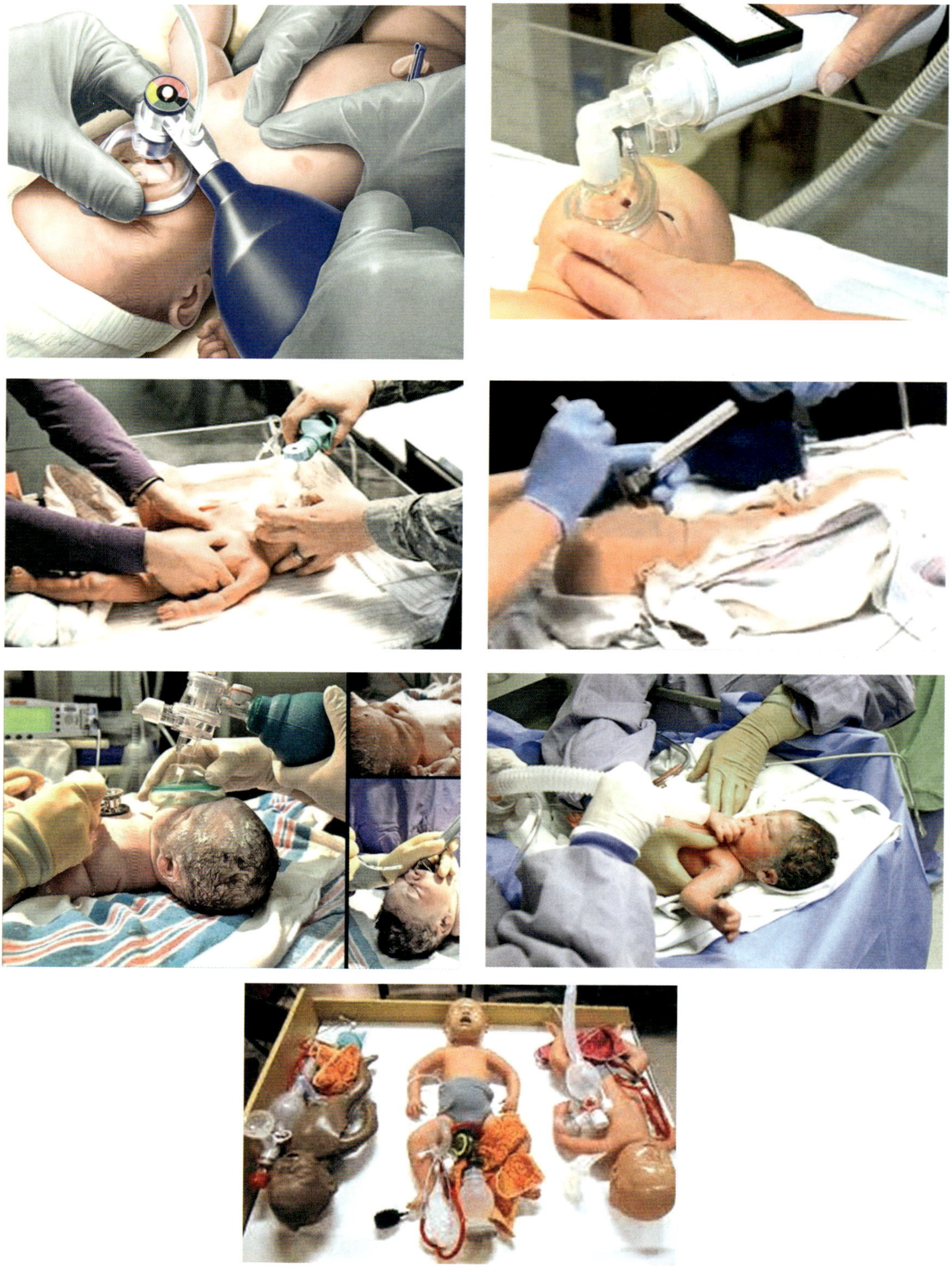

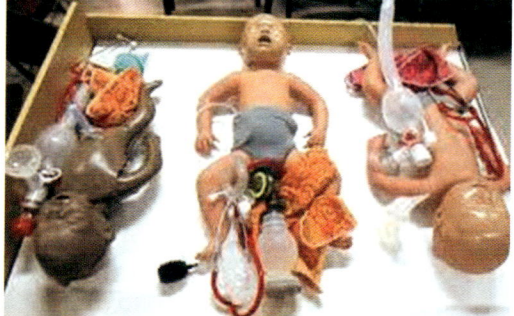

Fig. 24.1: Neonatal resuscitation

Miscellaneous

1. Radiant warmer
2. Stethoscope
3. Adhesive tape and bandage scissors
4. Syringe 1 ml, 2 ml, 5 ml and 20 ml sizes
5. Needles no 21, 22 and 26 G
6. Umbilical cord clamp
7. Gloves
8. Warm dry towel

Pre-procedure

1. Assess the Apgar score to know if resuscitation measures to be instituted.
2. Place infant under warmer, quickly dry off amniotic fluid, replace wet sheets with a dry one to prevent heat loss.
3. Place the baby on his back with slightly head down 15 degree tilt, neck slightly extended.
4. Suction the mouth first and then nose to clear airway passage
5. Give tactile stimulation if infant does not breath (flick or tap the sole of foot twice or rub the back), do not slap to bring spontaneous respiration
6. Check the vital signs, and color of the newborn which helps to determining further need for resuscitation.
7. *Note:* Evaluation should be done on respiration, heart rate and color. If the baby is apnoeic, heart rate is less then 100 bpm and central cyanosis is present, proceed for bag and mask ventilation or positive pressure ventilation.

BAG AND MASK VENTILATION/POSITIVE PRESSURE VENTILATION

Procedure

Place the newborn on his back with head slightly extended which helps in opening airway.

A tight seal is to be formed over the infant's mouth and nose with the face mask which prevents leakage of oxygen from the sides of the mask.

Ventilate at a rate of 40–50 per minute
Ventilate for 15–30 seconds and evaluate
Have an assistant to evaluate, listen to the heart rate for 6 seconds and multiply by 10.

Evaluation

1. If heart rate is above 100 bpm and spontaneous respirations are present, discontinue bagging
2. If heart rate is 60–100 bpm and increasing, continue ventilation, check weather chest is moving adequately
3. If heart rate is below 80 bpm, in addition to bagging and chest compressions, consider intubation and initiate medications
4. Signs of improvement, increasing heart rate, spontaneous respirations, improving color—continue to provide free flow oxygen by face mask after respirations are established.

If the baby deteriorates, check the following:
Placement of face mask for tight seal, head position and presence of secretions, presence of air in the stomach preventing chest expansion, oxygen being delivered (100% or not) for bagging lasting for more than two minutes insert an orogastric tube to vent the stomach.

What You Must Follow

Resuscitation

1. Check the responsiveness to call
2. Airway and cervical spine control.
   a. Assume that the cervical spine is damaged if there is any suspicion of injury above the clavicle keep a rigid cervical collar on
   b. Every poly trauma patient must receive 100% oxygen.
   c. Patient is talking—airway is adequate
   d. Patient unconscious—remove any liquid vomit's by suction.
   e. Remove any solid objects using Magill forceps.

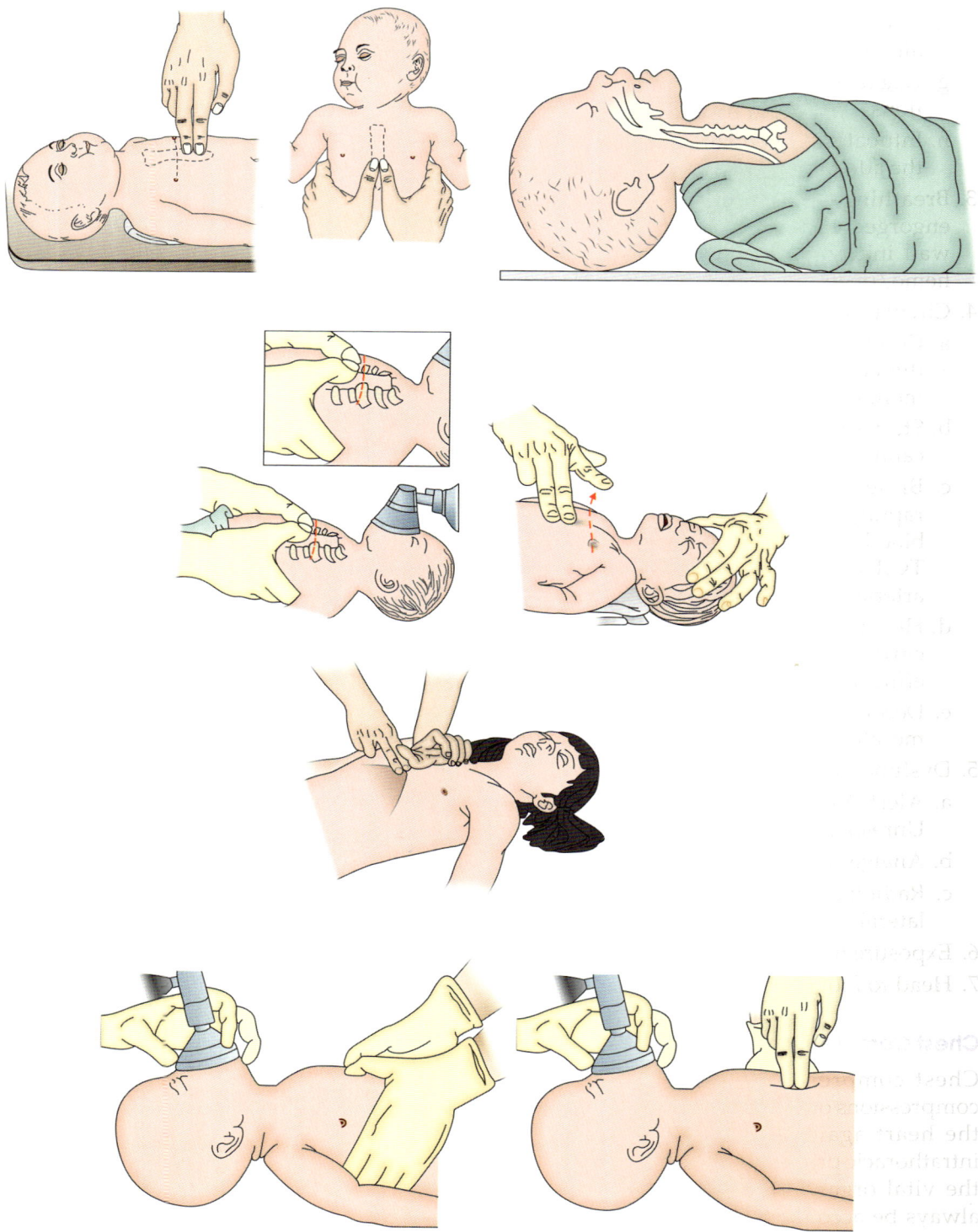

Fig. 24.2: Procedure to compress the chest with fingers

f. Put a nasopharyngeal/oropharengeal airway.

g. Gag reflex absent—endotracheal intubations

h. Intubate and ventilate if in doubts as to the adequacy of airway

3. Breathing—record respiratory rate and engorged veins in the neck, look for chest wall injury immediate chest drainage if hemo/pneumothorax

4. Circulation

a. Control any major external bleeds by direct pressure, Pulse, BP and cardiac monitor.

b. Start IV fluids through two 14 gauge cannula

c. BP less than 90 systolic-IL of colloid rapidly in the first instance, followed by blood and crystalloids as necessary Hb, TC,DC,Urea, electrolytes, X match, arterial blood gas analysis.

d. Heart sounds—muff bed consider-cardiac tamponade and pericardial effusion

e. Decompression by 16 G needle with ECG monitoring

5. Dysfunction neuro

a. Alert, Vocal response, Pain response, Unresponsive (AVPU)

b. Analgesia opiates IV + mettoclopramide

c. Radiological assessment cervical spine lateral

6. Exposure to injury assessment

7. Head to foot examination

Chest Compression

Chest compressions consist of rhythmic compressions of the sternum that compresses the heart against the spine increases the intrathoracic pressure and circulates blood to the vital organs. Chest compression must always be accompanied by ventilation with 100% oxygen to assure that the circulating blood is well oxygenated.

Indication

1. Heart rate less than 60 bpm after bagging with 100% oxygen for 15–30 seconds.

2. Heart rate 60–80 bpm and not increasing after bagging with 100% oxygen for 15–30 seconds.

Procedure

1. Compress the chest by placing the hands around the newborns chest with the fingers under the back to provide support and the thumbs over the lower third of the sternum (just above the xiphoid process) or use two fingers of one hand to compress the chest and place the other hand under the back to provide support.

2. Compress the sternum to a depth of approximately one-third of the antero-posterior diameter of the chest and with sufficient force to cause a palpable pulse. The fingers should remain in contact with the chest between compression.

3. Use three compression followed by one ventilation for a combined rate of compressions and ventilators of 120 each minute. This provides 90 compressions and 30 ventilations each minute. Pause for ½ second after every third compression for ventilation.

4. Check the heart rate after 30 seconds. If it is 60 bpm or more, discontinue compressions but continue ventilation until the heart rate is more than 100 bpm and spontaneous breathing (Note: If cardiac compression fails, endotracheal intubation should be initiated)

Endotracheal intubation: Indicated for heart rate below 60 per min in spite of bagging and chest compression. Presence of meconium in the amniotic fluid.

Procedure

1. Place infant with head slightly extended with a rolled towel under the shoulder.

2. Introduce laryngoscope over the baby tongue at the right corner of the mouth.

3. Advance 2–3 cm while rotating it to midline, until the epiglottis is seen. Evaluation of the epiglottis with the tip of the laryngoscope reveals the vocal cords

4. Suction secretions if needed

5. Pass the endotracheal tube a distance of 1.5–2 cm into the trachea, hold it firmly but gently in place and withdraw the laryngoscope slowly.

6. Attach the endotracheal tube to the adapter on the bag.

7. Ventilate with oxygen by bag. An assistant should check for adequate ventilation of both lungs with stethoscope.

Medications

Medications should be administered if despite adequate ventilation with 100% oxygen and chest compressions the heart rate remains at 80 bpm.

Recording

Record procedure in nurse's record, Document the baby's condition before and after procedure.

Using a handheld resuscitation bag and mask: If the patient is not breathing with an adequate rate and depth, or if the patient has lost the respiratory drive, a bag and mask may be used to deliver oxygen until the patient is resuscitated or can be intubated with an endotracheal tube. Bag and mask device AMBU bags (air mask bag unit) or BVMs (bag-valve-masks). The bags come in infant, pediatric, and adult size. The bag consists of an oxygen reservoir, oxygen tubing, the bag itself, a one way valve to prevent secretion from entering the bag, an exhalation port, an elbow, so that the bag can lie across the patients chest and a mask.

Research: New CPR matters could save lives in a heartbeat.

American students have designed a new mattress that can make cardiopulmonary resuscitation/CPR nearly twice as effective as an ordinary hospital mattress.

Before pushing, down to administer CPR is like pushing on a big sponge, which makes the force to go into the mattress, and not the body lying on it. But the new mattress has solved this problem, as it could be easily made firm by sucking the air out of the foam by just pushing a button.

It makes use of some tubing, a motor, and a vacuum pump, and takes just ten seconds to work. The researchers observed that only 43 percent of the CPR load winds up reaching the heart with the MTU students design, it leaps to 81% the students are now working to get this mattress into hospitals, especially in emergency rooms.

Chapter 25

Preoperative Checklist

1. Patients name
2. Age/sex
3. Reg. no., Bed no., Date
4. Surgeon and surgery

Anesthesia Record

1. Name of the patient, Bed no, Date
2. Surgeon
3. Anesthesiologist
4. Age, sex: M/F, wt in kg, Hb%, blood group
5. Started time, finished time
6. Other illness—DM, HT, IHD, MI, asthma, Kochs, Allergy, alcohol, tobacco, smoking
7. Previous SX
8. Investigation
9. Preoperative vital
10. ASA risk grade—I/II/II/IV/V=Emg/ Mid/Major/v. Maj/v.v.Maj
11. Types of anesthesia—regional; site, drug
12. Spinal/epidural—needle, drug
13. GA; induction—pentothal, prpofol, scoline, ketamine
14. Intubation; ET tube, cuff/pack
15. Maintenance; O_2/N_2O/halothane/trilene/ isoflurane/sevoflurane
16. Relaxant; tracurium/pavlon
17. Short GA; drug
18. Position;supine/prone/spica/litho-tomic/lateral

19. Postoperative; reversal; atropine/glycol-p-mg/neostigmine-mg
20. Vital; BP, pulse, SaO_2 urine output
21. Conscious/drowsy/unconscious/ extubated
22. Ryles tube, Foley catheter, cavfafix, veinflow
23. Atropine, emset/perinom, fortwin/ phenergan, lasix/deriphyllin, trmadol/ diclofenac

Request for Histopathology/Culture

1. Date
2. Age, IPD no
3. Sex: M/F
4. Specimen
5. Clinical diagnosis
6. Nature of tissue and site of origin
7. Duration of disease
8. Lymph nodes draining the area
9. Radiological finding
10. LMP (if gynae specimen)
11. Relevant clinical notes
12. Referred by

Autoclave register: Stick sigma strips, date, start time, stop time door opening, description of items, operated by, inspected by *Fumigation activity register* date, TO, solution used, start time, stop time, pre swab test application, swab test result, corrective action if swab test +ve, conducted by, verified by Matron sign

Patients case sheet	Ward Yes/no	OT Yes/no	Ward Yes/no
Patients vitals—TPR, BP, Weight			
Consent			
Patient NMB SINCE			
Any allergy			
Investigation			
USG			
ECG			
ECHO			
X-ray			
CT			
MRI			
Doppler			
Latest HB			
H/O DM Latest FBS			
Blood group			
Blood arranged			
Any other reports			
Operation site shaved and cleaned			
General hygiene is maintained			
Dentures removed/loose teeth			
Jewellery/nail polish/contact lenses removed			
Voided/transportation			
Premedication-time			
1.			
2.			
3.			
Bed sheet			
Gown/pant, shirt			
Advanced Rs.			
In charge signature and remarks	Ward nurse sign	TO nurse sign	Ward nurse sign

Intraoperative Nurses Notes, Description and Sign

      Date

      Time   Postoperative assessment by RMO

                                Surgeon

                                Name of the surgery

Anesthetists, anesthesia used

Condition of patient when received in ICU/Ward

G/C, TPRR, BP

SAO_2, P/A

RS, CNS

CVS

Check for drain/catheter/dressing/cast, etc.

Position of the patient, NBM

Postoperative medications

Description of the operation performed in the month of—medium, major, total.

GI endoscope department consent, e.g. I have been informed the need and nature or procedure and its advantage and disadvantages. I am aware that this procedure may need mild sedation and if necessary, a biopsy will be done.

MISCELLANEOUS

Morning Duty in TO

1. Daily morning sweeping and moping inside and outside
2. Carbonization done by staff-autoclave room
3. Fold all doctors' clothes and kept in locker.
4. Kept footwear on stand
5. Checked the oxygen, nitrous, CO_2 cylinders
6. Empty the waste products
7. Evening duty—check to before surgery, operation entry done in computer, get all the clean linen from laundry, prepare set for next day, autoclave all instruments and linen, carbolize again, prepare dressing materials according to number of cases (gauze, gamji pad, gamji roll, rollers pack, linen, etc.) arrange the staff for next days duty.
8. In case any night emergency inform supervisor
9. Fumigate to every alternate day

To Registers Maintained

1. Delivery register
2. Autoclave
3. Fumigation
4. Hydrocele
5. MTP
6. ECT
7. Endoscopy appointments
8. Purchase book of pharmacy
9. Medicine entry

Consent for Surgery (Diagnostic/Therapeutic Procedures)

- The nature and extent of the procedure to be performed and risk involved, even those, which unlikely to occur involve serious consequences.
- Alternative procedure and methods of treatment
- The dangers and probable consequences of such alternative
- The estimated period of hospitalization or incapacity and the estimated period of convalescence
- The expected consequences of the procedure upon my future health
- I understand that these are risks, such as the risks of into other serious complications, in the preoperative and postoperative stages of my care, which can result in serious consequences such as loss of the use of parts of my body and life.
- If nurse reads and understands to how important it is to give explanation, not rushing to get singer, each hospital has there policy of content format medical risk, anesthetic risk.
- I have asked all of the questions, which I thought, were important in deciding whether to undergo treatment or diagnosis. Those questions have been answered to my satisfaction.
- I understand that no assurance can be given that the procedure will be successful or no guarantee or warranty of success or cure has been given to me.
- I have been advised that I may have anesthesia which is rare instances has serious and even fatal complications.
- I further authorize and request my physical and his associate assistants and appropriate hospital personnel to perform such additional procedure, which in their judgment are incidentally necessary or appropriate hospital personnel to perform

such additional procedure that in their judgment are incidentally necessary or appropriate to carry art my diagnosis/ treatment.

- I have been afforded the opportunity to consult with other physician to my complete satisfaction before signing this form and I understand that I have the right to refuse any medical and surgical procedures and treatment.
- I authorize the hospital to dispose of or use for research any tissue or a body part that may be necessary to remove it's a manner consistent with regulation.
- I read and fully understand the above consent stated and this consent was given.

Chapter 26

Medical and Surgical Instruments

Instruments commonly used in antiseptic preparations are sponge holding forceps, towel clips and Moynihan's tetra-forceps.

Ideal *scalp* should be light, the blade should be fairly sharp, the handle should give a good grip and have movements like a swinging cut, it should have straight back, sterilization should be not a problem.

Scissors are classified according to curvature or angles, according to points or tips, according to use. Sterilization by autoclaving, as boiling affects the sharpness of the instruments.

Sutures are classified as absorbable (natural and synthetic) and non-absorbable. Ideal absorbable suture should be perfectly sterilized, should not be absorbed prematurely, should be flexible and should possess satisfactory knot pull tensile strength. Catgut is available as plain which has a duration of one week and chromic about two to three weeks duration.

Stainless steel wires are used chiefly in bone sutures, Thiersch's operation for rectal prolapsed in children, etc.

Surgical needles classified according to shapes (straight and curved) according to cutting edge (round body) according to its eye (triangular tipped and round tipped needles) according to its use.

Surgical diathermy is a high frequency electric current, produced from a special machine. Machine has mains switch, foot pedal, active electrode, passive electrode and coagulating and cutting dials.

There are two varieties of tissue and dissecting forceps—toothed and un-toothed.

Instruments are sharp, blunt, plastic, glasswares, enamel, steel, etc.

Preparation of the Theater Equipment and Supplies

Cleaning

1. Instrument must be thoroughly washed, either by hand or by using a sonic washer
2. Particular care should be paid to joints and grooves and delicate instruments such as those used in ophthalmic surgery must be carefully handled
3. All instruments should be soaked regularly in a lubricating

Disposable syringes are generally used, but glass syringes are used they should be thoroughly cleaned and packed with the piston and barrel separate.

Packing

In prepacked sets, instruments are prepared on a metal tray which is covered by a large drape which is secured to a rim on the tray

1. Swabs and drapes may also be included in this pack, depending on local policy.
2. The drape is then folded over the trays the set is double rapped in waterproof paper.

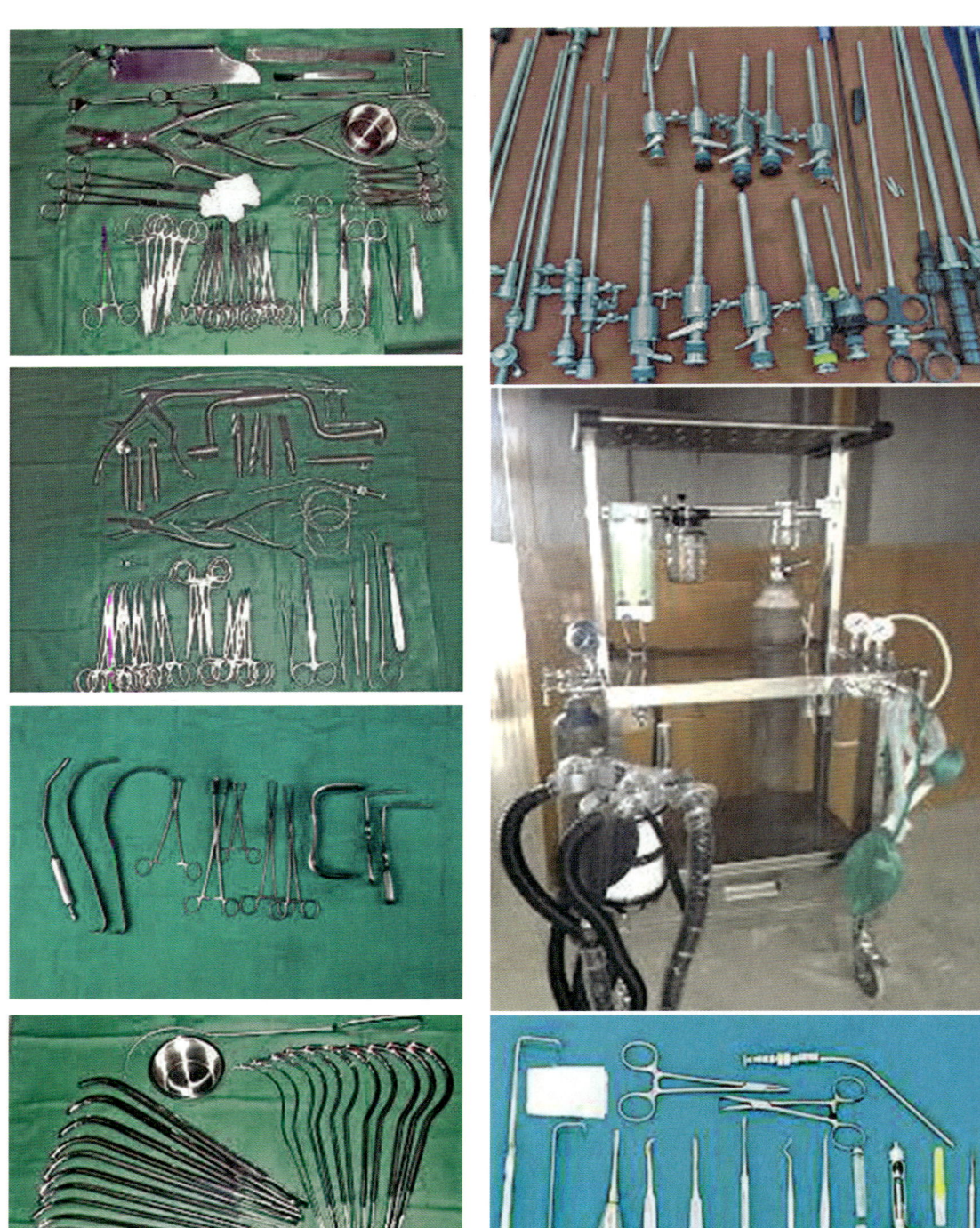

Fig. 26.1: Surgical instruments

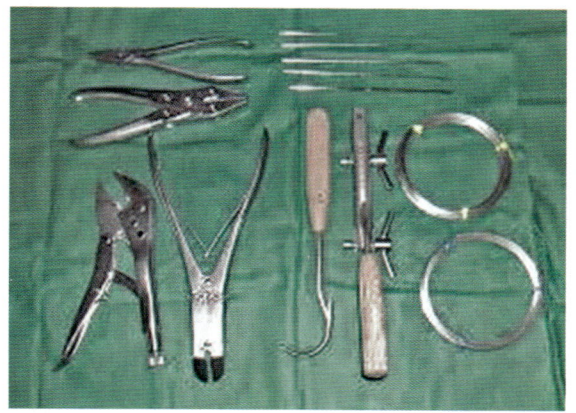
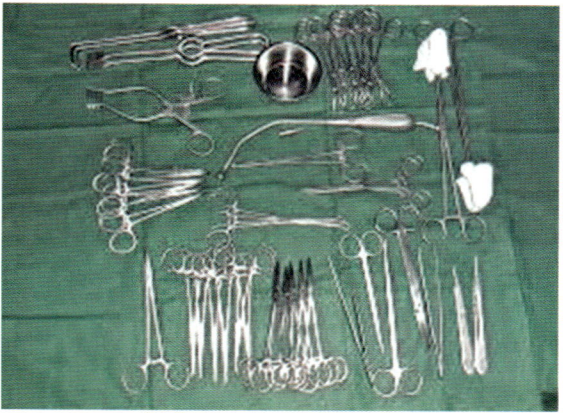
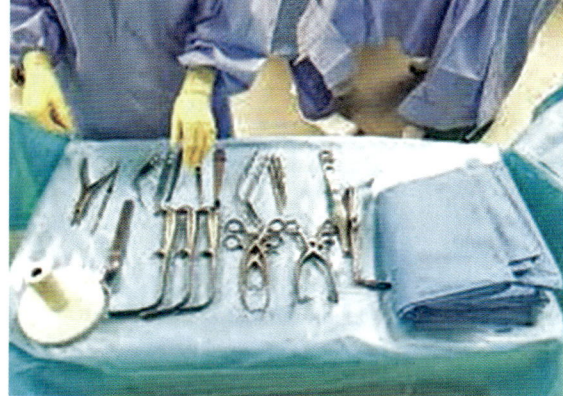
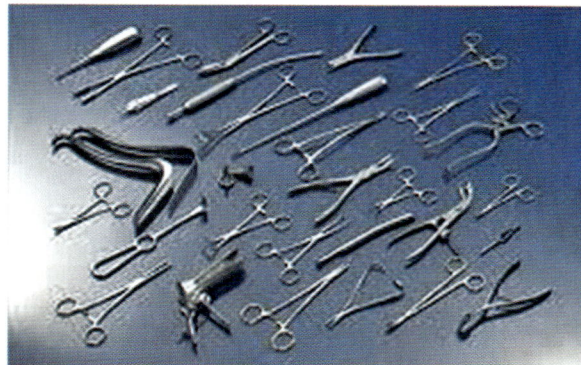

Fig. 26.2: Surgical instruments and equipment

3. Autoclave tape is applied and the set is lightly tied.
4. The same principles are used when preparing metal ware and drapes for sterilization.
5. It is done by CSSD staff

6. Instruments can be autoclaved in perforated metal tins which a new wrapped in the same way as instrument sets.
7. Swabs, dressing an gloves are brought commercially and disposable.
8. All swabs used for surgical contain a radio-opaque marker.

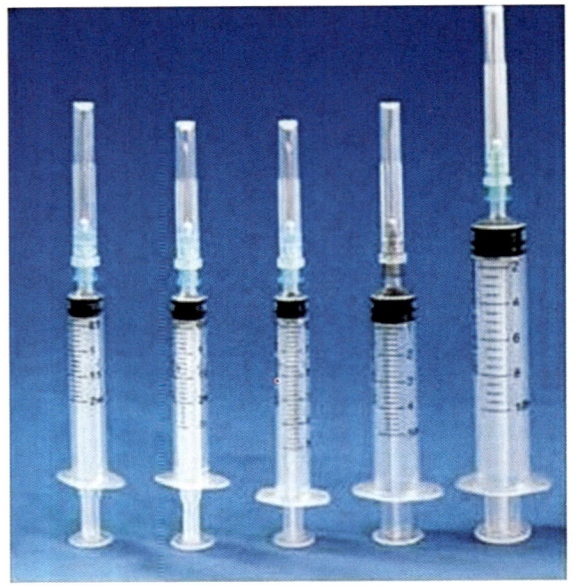
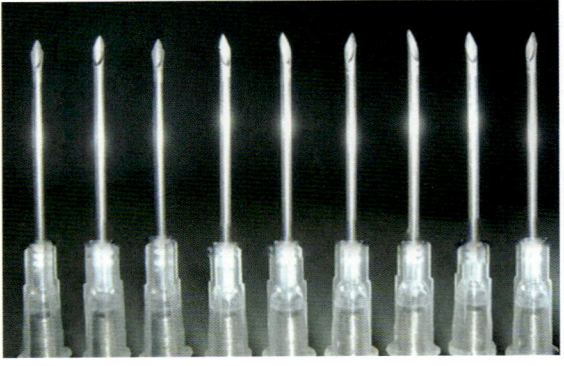
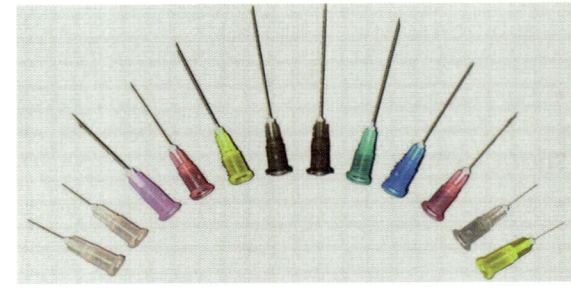
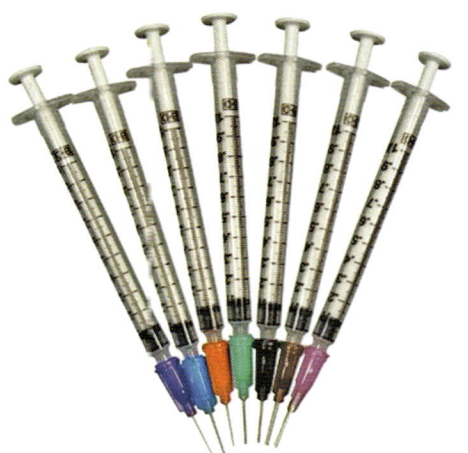
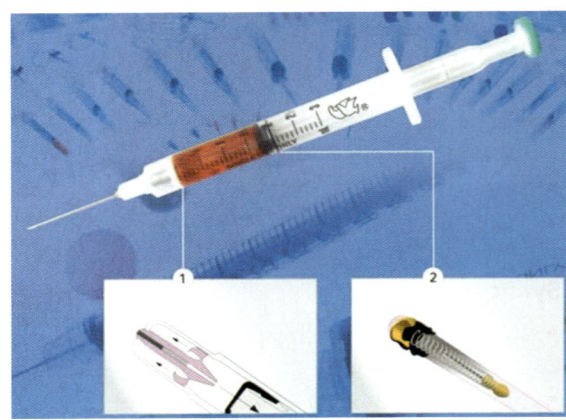
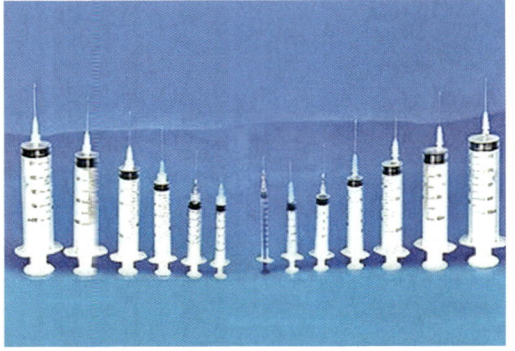

Fig. 26.3: Different size needles and syringes

Instruments

- Always wash the used instruments in 0.5% of chloride solution for 5 min.
- Wash the instrument in cold running water.
- Separate sharp instruments form blunt and a instruments.
- Put rubber cap on tine-tip instruments.
- Dry them thoroughly.
- Make different pack, wrapping them.
- Autoclaving
- Mingled instrument must be kept open.
- Decontaminate all needles attached to syringe and flush with 0.5% chloride solution sodium hypochlorite immediately after use.
- Send stainless needle for autoclaving.

Sharp Instruments

- Under solution Lysol 2% glutaraldehyde for 20–30 minutes protoscope and broncho-scope
- Pull out abrader from the scope.
- Immune obdurate and speculum in 0.5% chlorine solution minimum for 10 minutes.
- Remove both item and rinse in cold water and then wash in soap water stream.
- Boil for 10 min
- Pull and send the scrape for autoclaving.

Syringe

- Wash thoroughly pack and send for autoclaving
- Needles should not be kept in contact with glass syringe.
- Preston and barrel are kept separately into some back rubbing.

EXAMPLES OF TRAY SET-UP IN OT

I and D Tray Instruments—I and II

1. Gally cup	(01)
2. Sinus forceps	(01)
3. Suction tip	(01)
4. Scoop	(01)
5. Straight mosquito	(02)
6. Mosquito forceps	(02)
7. Artery forceps	(02)
8. Allies forceps	(02)
9. Scissor set with needle holder	(02)
10. Tooth and nontooth forceps	(01)
11. BP handle number	4-1-3-1
12. Sponge holder	(01)

Craniotomy Tray

1. Tray	
2. Gally cup	04
3. BP handle	No-3, 2, 4, 1
4. Addison tooth	01
5. Adhisoon nontooth	
6. Normal tooth	01
7. Normal nontooth	01
8. Long Addison tooth	01
9. Artery forceps	06
10. St. artery forceps	15
11. St. mosquito	06
12. Side artery	15
13. Long artery	02
14. Scissor St. big	
15. Scissor stilly big	
16. Needle holder	03
17. Towel clip	8 big, 4 small
18. Mosquito forceps	06
19. Allies forceps	05
20. Sponge holder	
21. Suction tip adaptor-04	(2 sets)
22. Periostium-03, small	01
23. Dissector (different sizes)	07
24. Diamond forceps	01
25. Mastoid retractor	02
26. Injection tray with soft role	
27. Plain forceps (bipolar type)	02
28. Long fine tooth and nontooth One each	
29. Normal long tooth	
30. Disc forceps	03
31. Brain retractor	04

32. Right angle retractor   One pair
33. Nerve hook   01
34. Gigli passer   01
35. Gigli wire   Two
36. Tumar forceps   01

AV Fistula Tray

1. Sponge holder   01
2. Artery forceps   03
3. Mosquito forceps   03
4. Needle holder   01
5. BP handle   No 3-2
6. Buldocks clamps   03
7. Addison tooth-02 and nontooth   02
8. Hydrodisection canulla   01
9. Micro instrument
10. Tying forceps   03
11. Micro tooth forceps   01
12. Needle holder   01
13. Small scissors   04
14. Small mosquito   03
15. Gally cup   02
16. Towel clip   02
17. Cats paw-one pair
18. Suture cutting scissor   01

Piles Set

1. Artery forceps   6
2. Allies forceps   6
3. Mosquito forceps   4
4. Kidney tray   1
5. Probe   6
6. Proctoscope   2
7. Self retaining retracter   1
8. Gallycup with needle pack   1
9. Speculum   2
10. One side speculum   4
11. BP handle no. 4 (1) 1 no. 3 . 1
12. Sponge holder   1
13. Scoope   1
14. Towel clip   2
15. Set of scissors with needle holder
16. Tooth + nontooth forceps   1 each
17. Badcock   2

HSG Set

1. Sim's speculum   1
2. Valsalum   1
3. Artery forceps   1
4. Sponge holder   1
5. Allies forcep   1
6. RT canula   1

Septoplasty

1. Nasal speculum   1
2. Periosteum   2
3. Packing forcep—1, small—1
4. Nasal speculum   7
5. Chisel   4
6. Elevator Rt. Lf   4
7. Hammer   1
8. A pair of scissors   1

Tympanoplasty

1. Cup of forceps   2
2. Side dressing forcep   1
3. A pair of scissors   2
4. Circle knife   1
5. Sickle knife   1
6. Boll probe   1
7. Hook   1
8. Micro pick   1
9. Mastoid rectractor   1

Tonsillectomy

1. BP handle no. 7   1
2. Adenoid forcep   1
3. Adenoid rectractor   1
4. Mouth gauge   1
5. Luck's forceps   1
6. Tonsilar snace   1
7. Long artery forceps–2,   st–1
8. A pair of scissors   1
9. Long tooth forceps   1
10. Towel clip   2
11. Tongue depressor   2
12. Kidney tray   1
13. Gally cup   1

14. Suction tip	1
15. Suction nozzle	1
16. Gauze pieces	20
17. Linen no. 40	10 pieces

Laminectomy

1. Periosteum big   1
2. Disc forceps different size (St, up, down)
3. Circle scoop (different size)
4. Nerve root
5. Spine cutter
6. Spine Nibbler
7. Clovad's retracter (cervical)
8. Cervical spreder
9. Self retaining
10. Parch (up cut 2, down cut)

Plastic Surgery Set

1. Skin books	2
2. Cat's paws	2
3. Fine forceps tooth	2
4. Fine forceps nontooth	2
5. A pair of scissors short curved	1
6. A pair of scissors long curved	1
7. A pair of scissors short straight	1
8. A pair of scissors long straight	1
9. Micro mosquito forceps	1
10. Towel clips	2

D and C Set

1. Dilators (all size)	15
2. Uterine sound	1
3. Valselum	1
4. Uterine curettes	2 (short, blunt)
5. Ovum forceps	1
6. Sim's forceps	1
7. Suction conulla	2
8. AV retractor	1
9. Sponge holder	1

Cut Down Tray

1. Sponge holder	1
2. Small mosquito	3

3. St mosquito	4
4. Allies forceps	4
5. Needle holder	2
6. Fine scissors	2
7. Stillies	1
8. Addison forceps	1 pair
9. Hook	1
10. Gally cup with needle pack	

Extra for Laparotomy

1. Diver's retractor	3 (small, medium, large)
2. Doyen's retractor	4 (all size)
3. Right angle retractor large	1 pair
4. Sponge holding forceps long	1
5. Robert's clamps	3
6. Malleable retractor long	1
7. Self retaining abdominal retractor	1
8. Intestinal crushing clamp	2
9. Long artery forceps	3

Urology

1. Big kidney tray	1
2. Gally cup	2
3. Sponge holder	1
4. Artery	1
5. A pair of scissors	1
6. Towel clip	1

Extra Instrument Tray

1. Rt. angle retractor 1"	2 pairs
2. Long stills scissors	1
3. Sponge holders	2
4. Mixter forceps	3
5. Long artery	3
6. Kocker's clamp	1
7. St. artery	1
8. St. mosquito	1
9. Yonke's (throat) suction	1

A Major Set

1. Sponge holder	03
2. Mosquito forceps	06

3. Artery forceps — 12
4. Babcock small — 02
5. Allies forceps — 06
6. St. moscuito — 05
7. St. cocker — 05
8. Big artery — 05
9. Big St. artery — 05
10. Big babcock — 02
11. Very big artery — 02
12. Big allies — 04
13. Scissor set and small stille — 01
14. Needle holder — 03
15. Mixter forceps — 03
16. Occlusion clamp — 02
17. St. occlusion clamp — 04
18. "Cv" shape — 02
19. Big tooth and nontooth — 01 each
20. Broad forceps — 01
21. BP handle no. — 3,2,4,1
22. Towel clip-06 (Mayo)
23. Kidney tray big and small — 01 each
24. Gally cup with needle pack
25. Suction tip — 01
26. Suction tube — 01
27. Normal tooth and nontooth — 01 each

Chapter 27

Infection Control Nurse

Infection control nurses, sometimes-called infection prevention nurses, help prevent patient infections in hospitals and clinics. They instruct other nurses and health care staff on proper sanitation procedures; they also study patients' bacteria to identify any infections that may have possibly resulted from a patient's health care. Infection control nurses are usually the ones responsible for notifying the closest branch of the Centers for Disease Control. Things you would do

1. Instruct nurse for proper hand washing procedures
2. Create sanitation plans
3. Study patients bacterial plans

Your job characteristics
1. Patient facing
2. Managerial
3. Research-orientated

Infection Control and Prevention

About 10% of people in hospital acquire an infection, although this figure may be higher for people with low immune systems or people in intensive care units.

What do infection and colonization mean?

An infection, in general terms, is the illness caused by the growth of a germ on or in a person.

Sometimes the infection does not give any symptoms—this is called an 'asymptomatic' infection.

When the germ is commonly found on our body without causing an illness, we call it carriage or colonization.

Carriage may be very short term (transient). For example, acquired by touching someone but quickly removed by washing your hands, or persistent with the germ multiplying on your body (usually called colonization).

In certain circumstances, the germs that colonise in our bodies may go on to give an infection.

What sort of infections is there and how do they spread?

Infections can range from the minor, like coughs and colds, to more serious ones like septicemia (blood poisoning) and wound infections. Infections tend to be more common for people in hospital because they are in close contact with other patients and staff who themselves may be colonised or suffering infection.

Infections can spread quickly unless certain measures are taken. Any patient who has an operation or other procedure where the skin is broken, like intravenous infusions, is at risk of infection.

Patients with certain conditions are also more at risk from infection. For instance, those with heart, kidney or skin diseases or those with low immune systems. Other patients at risk include very young babies or children who are not feeding well.

The germs that cause infection spread in various ways, the main methods being:

- *Airborne:* The air, such as the chickenpox virus, carries the germs.
- *Droplet spread:* Infectious droplets of moisture are coughed or breathed out during infection. They settle on surfaces and may be transferred to another person's eyes or mouth, usually by their hands.
- *Direct contact:* By touching someone that has the infection, such as scabies.
- *Indirect contact:* By contact with dirty equipment or other materials.

There are various ways we can all prevent infections, some of which are outlined below.

MONITORING

What can we do?

When a new member of staff joins the hospital, they are checked for immunity against certain diseases and immunized if needed. They are also screened using a questionnaire, or by testing, to see if they are carrying certain infections. If necessary, we can then treat them.

When a child is admitted to hospital, we always ask for a swab of their nose and throat and a sample of faeces. This is then sent to the laboratory and checked for germs that are resistant to antibiotics. When the results are available, this helps the doctors and nurses decide if any special precautions are needed to prevent cross infection. If the child is carrying a germ that is resistant to the common antibiotics, then we will nurse them in a single cubicle and alert this on the computer that contains your child's information.

What you can do?

You can help by telephoning outpatients or the ward before you come in if your child has been in contact with any infectious disease, like chickenpox or a tummy bug, so we can prevent it spreading to other children and their families.

HAND WASHING

What we can do?

Everyone being exposed to your child, like doctors, nurses, members of staff and yourself, should wash their hands thoroughly before and after they touch your child. This is a good way of reducing health care acquired infection.

We provide liquid soap and water on every ward. Alcohol gel can be used to wash hands quickly if they are not physically dirty.

What you can do?

You can help by asking members of staff being exposed to your child whether they have washed their hands. You should also ask your visitors to wash their hands, and make sure your hands are clean too. Remember that alcohol gel is available as well as soap and water.

With bad hand hygiene—identified as the biggest contributor to the almost 2 million hospital acquired infection that kill 1 lakh people every year. The hospitals there are testing a new wristband monitor that reminds doctors to wash their hands. When they enter the patients room. It gives a buzzing signal to wash hands; it also sets off further warning if the cleaning is not up to the mark. A good hand wash should last at least 15 seconds. Researchers say our hands probably carry at least 3000 different bacteria belonging to move then 100 species many are not pathogens but a few can set off feco-oral diarrhea, fever viral, skin infections, common cold. You would never know what damage unclean hands can cause your health.

ENVIRONMENT

What we can do?

We try to make sure that all areas of the hospital are clean. Each ward has a housekeeper who monitors how clean the ward is and takes action to get an area cleaned if necessary. We work closely with our domestics who work very hard to maintain our high standards of cleanliness.

We realize that sometimes we do not manage to reach our high standards. However, the senior nurses, managers and infection control team all try to resolve any problems quickly.

We also have special 'clean' cubicles for children who are severely immune-suppressed. For instance patients who have recently had a bone marrow transplant.

On very rare occasions, a ward may need to be closed because of an outbreak of infection such as diarrhea and vomiting. If this happens, we will inform you as quickly as possible as we may need to restrict access to the ward.

What you can do?

You can help by telling us if you think an area is not clean enough. You can also keep the area by your child's bed clear of waste, like dirty cups, used tissues and leftover food, and toys tidied away when they are not being used. There is limited storage space by each bed, please use it to keep belongings out of the way.

Each bed area is cleaned once a day between 10.30 am and 4.30 pm. As space is limited, please go to the parents' room while it is being cleaned. Cleaning should take about 20 minutes. If the bed area is kept tidy then it is easier for our domestics to clean.

If you have any questions please talk to the ward housekeeper.

If a ward is closed due to infection, please keep your movements within the hospital to a minimum and avoid visiting other wards if possible. If possible, you should also restrict the number of people visiting your child and let us know if a visitor develops any signs of infection once they have returned home.

EQUIPMENT

What we can do?

All our equipment, like infusion pumps and ventilators, is cleaned regularly, decontaminated in between patients and maintained to make sure it is working well. Every member of staff who is trained to use the equipment is also trained to report if the equipment fails or needs cleaning.

What you can do?

You can help by telling us if you think a piece of equipment is not working properly. All external parts of equipment should be cleaned regularly, so if you think it needs cleaning, please tell the ward housekeeper.

PROTECTIVE CLOTHING

What we can do?

Our staff will wear an apron and gloves if there is a risk of contact with:

- Bodily fluids, like saliva, blood, vomit, urine (wee) or faeces (poo)
- Patients colonised or infected with germs such as MRSA

Latex-free gloves are available if your child is allergic to latex.

We advise our staff to wear masks if there is a risk of breathing in an infection. In certain circumstances, where there is a risk of bodily fluids being splashed into the eyes and mouth, we recommend our staff wear a visor or goggles.

What we can do?

You can help by telling us when your child is admitted if they have had any infections with germs like MRSA, hepatitis B or C, or HIV. It will not make any difference to the quality of

diarrhoea and vomiting, a rash or wound infection, we will take samples of urine, faeces, wound swabs and blood.

These samples will be sent to the laboratory to see if they can identify whether your child has an infection or not.

While the samples are being checked, and afterwards if your child has an infection, they will be nursed in a cubicle on their own, or along with other children with the same infection. The staff will wear protective clothing, like aprons and gloves while caring for your child.

We will continue to take samples regularly, to check whether your child still has the infection.

What happens if my child is or becomes infected or colonized with MRSA or other antibiotic resistant organisms in hospital?

If the child is carrying a germ that is resistant to common antibiotics then we will nurse them in a single cubicle and alert this on the computer that contains your child's information.

We will inform you if we think this has been acquired while in hospital and we will investigate every situation to detect the possible risk factors so they can be reduced.

More Information

If you have any questions about infections or infection control, please ask to speak to the nurse in charge or the infection control link nurse for your ward or unit.

Chapter 28

Understanding Nursing Profession and New Research in Surgery

Surgery is advancing very fast, and the surgeons are always confronted with a barrage and changing information from the old fundamentals to the new concepts.

A surgical patient is both healthy and fit except for some surgical problems that needs operative treatment or in a bad condition due to advanced surgical diseases.

Science has made rapid progress over the past decades. Much of our comforts in life are a direct result of these scientific discoveries. The meaning of the terms science and technology have changed significantly from one generation to another. Both science and technology imply a thinking process, pure sciences have made many practical as well as theoretical contributions. Science has proved to be great help to mankind in medical and surgical field.

The human body is incredibly complex and intricate system, one that never ceases to amaze:

1. 500 g fat = 11 km blood vessels. When you gain 500 mg of fat, your body makes 11 km of blood vessels. This means your body must work harder to pump blood through all of these extra new vessels, straining your heart. Fortunately, if you lose 500 gm you body will break down and re-absorb the now unnecessary vessels.

2. It is hard to grasp just how small the atoms that make up your body are until you look at the sheer number of them. An adult is made up of around 7,000,000,000,000,000,000,000,000,000,000 (7 octillion) atoms (1 octillion = 1000 trillion trillion)

3. Larger molecule? chromosome 1—a normal human cell has 23 pairs of chromosomes in its nuclei, each a single, very long molecule of DNA chromosome 1 is the biggest to pack in the amount of information that is encoded in the molecule.

4. Our digestive acids are strong enough to dissolve zinc. But cells in the stomach lining renew so quickly that the acids do not have time to dissolve it.

5. The focusing muscles of the eyes move around 100.000 times a day. To give your leg muscles the same workout, you would need to walk 80 km every day. Do not even think about it.

6. Human bone is as strong as granite in supporting weight. 8.6 tones that is how much one cubic inch of bone can support. That is four times as much as concrete can support.

7. The skin is the largest organ in the body. In an adult person it covers about 20 sq ft. if constantly flakes away, each person sheds around 18 kg in a lifetime.

8. 640.000 is the number of sense receptors, scattered unevenly over the body's surface. These receptors are most abundant in the ridges of the fingertips, in the lips, at the tip of the tongue in the palms, and on the soles of the feet.

9. In movies, a human body explodes if it is pushed into space without suit. But it is mostly fiction. Although liquids do boil in a vacuum, your blood is kept under pressure by your circulatory system and would be just fine. It is lack of air that will kill you.

10. You are sleep deprived if you fall asleep within 5 minutes of hitting the sack. The idea is between 10 and 15 minutes, meaning you are still tired enough to sleep deeply, but not so exhausted you feel sleepy during the day.

To ensure quality clinical practice, nursing education has to visualize the modern trends in nursing specially consumers rights, health information system, ethical legal obligation of nurses, evidence based practice renewal of registration, specialization in nursing, independent nurse practice, concept of globalization through exchange programme.

Florence Nightingale

Nursing is an act and if it is to be made an art, it requires as exclusive as devotion, as hard as preparation, as any painter's or sculptors work, for what is the having to do with dead canvas or cold marble. Compared with having to do with the living body, the temple of God's spirit? It is love of the fine arts, I had almost said, the finest of the fine arts.

The nurse should have real desire and willingness to work hard. They have to realize the hardship of the predecessors who worked hard for the development of the profession.

There may be instances where nurses may get discouraged, dissatisfied and rebuked. In all these occasions, they have to maintain as emotional balance. When they are upright with their dealing with patients and others, they can be proud of that they have done their

part well. Whenever they may be, their aim must be to work hard for the welfare of humanity. They have to develop the questioning mind to acquire more knowledge and to achieve their aim so that they are able to think logically and approach scientifically. Technological development widens their ways. Aim should be patient get benefit and health promotion venture.

Nursing care is always arranged around, or fitted into, the physician's therapeutic plan.

Nursing is an art to be cultivated and a profession to be followed.

Nursing has passed through many phases. Theses changes were necessary to meet the changing needs of the society. The art of healing began 1000 years ago with the primitive man trying to provide relief in sickness and suffering motivated by feelings of sympathy and kindness. Team approach was used to treat the sick person. The physician directed the treatment, the nurse carried out the care, the pharmacist prepared the medicine and the spiritual care was administered along with these.

During the last quarter of a century, a profound change has taken place in the work of nurses. Some diseases that were once incurable have yielded to new medical and surgical advances, some that used to run a prolonged course are speedily controlled, others that necessitated hospital care can now be treated at home. This was involved widening our horizons new techniques, new operations to be assisted. The teacher must ensure that the methods she is advocating are not only sound in theory, but are the most effective and acceptable in practice.

There is often a great variance between the way the nurse learned to do process in the classroom and the way she practices them in the ward. This variance may be due to lack of enough of the right kind of patient care equipped, pressure of work, or it may be due to the nurse's inability to plan or lack of initiative and imagination to improve or to determine what comes first in a ward service. Service to humankind is the primary function of nurses and the reason for the existence of the nursing profession. Need for nursing service is universal.

Nursing procedure should be scientifically sound. Interchange of information among agencies insures better relationship procedures; system of operation policies governing nursing practice should be; evaluated, reviewed and revised at regularly planned intervals.

Principles

- Every physically ill person is potentially and emotionally upset person.
- Illness causes the patient to become dependent with a consequent threat to his inner, personal security. He often becomes the victim of fears and fantasies and it is harder for him to recognize and manage his feelings.
- His emotional needs must be met before the patient will be ready to accept help.
- The nurse must be aware of her own emotional needs to avoid over including the patient or satisfying her own need to feel important at the expense of the patient.
- Citizens of a country look to a hospital as a safe haven for treatment and recovery from illness.

Initiative of INC

1. PHD nursing curriculum has been developed.
2. Minimum standards of nursing practice have been developed.
3. Code of ethics has been formulated
4. Pilot project on quality assurance
5. Model (CAM) implementation in selected wards at PGI.
6. Data base of nursing education.
7. Student patient ratio has been relaxed for 1:5 to 1:3
8. Qualification and experience of nursing teachers has been relaxed to 2012.
9. Sharing of teaching faculty for both diploma an graduate programme.
10. Age increased for teaching faculty up to 70 years.

Nurses spend most of their time with the patient and generally share more meaningful relationship with them. Nurses being in unique position need to provide the highest quality to care with minimal risk to patients. The concept of quality in health car in has being increasingly appreciated and in the last few years, health care providers have recognized that survival and competitiveness are essential to improve patent out come, she needs to ask herself.

What is a quality care?
How is to be delivered?
How it can be measured?

Answer: Nurses need to redesign the work culture, re-teach specific skills. These are no short cuts to quality, it is ongoing continuous process of improvement in order to improve quality practice, innovation, prevention of error, self-development are essentially elements to be incorporated in the total good practices. Improvement is always possible care is done in right way. Nurses should accept quality as an integral part of their role. Harboring; fear is not an effective motivator, therefore they must enhance their knowledge, widen there practice base, and transform their beliefs and attitudes quality care is difficult to measure, understand and motor because of many variables like types of health care (acute care, home care, primary care, long term care, medical and surgical care) patient receive care in number of setting.

Migration of Nurses

Nursing is a service-oriented job combined with a sense of compassion and commitment. Care is directed to whole person, not just the body part. To be called a nurse is an honor because we work with human beings life and death. From vital parameters at admission until discharge she handles from hand washing until tracheotomy care from hygienic care until medication all work, she does at bedside of the patients. Delivering a child till resuscitation of a child. Where do they work? Why do people options for nursing? Nursing has good career options, it is an never ending process, due to increasing population there is a great scope to go higher. 2020 there will be 800.000 shortages of nurses in the world.

There is following nursing scope for higher education such as:

1. Academic nursing education
2. Admission nursing
3. Aerospace nursing
4. Ambulatory care nursing
5. Business and marketing nursing
6. Clinic nursing
7. Emergency nursing
8. Employee health nursing
9. Epidemiological nursing
10. Forensic nursing
11. Hospice nursing
12. Infection control nurses
13. Legal nurse
14. Military
15. Navy
16. Air force
17. Information
18. Psychologist
19. Research
20. Office nurses
21. Evidence based practice nurses anesthetic
22. Oncological
23. Neonatal
24. Admission
25. OB Gyn
26. Ophthalmic
27. Preoperative
28. Orthopedic
29. Radiological
30. Rehabilitator
31. School nurse
32. Travel nurse
33. So she gets optimal level of functioning

Migration of high skilled nurse from less developed nation to developed nation is inevitable part of the process of globalization and this process has positive and negative aspect. Pull and push factors—health in an industry professional developing, promotional opportunities, working conditions, that time nurses change where by changing the job she gets the opportunity and financial security.

Unmanaged migration reasons are:

1. Shortage of nurses in the country
2. Declined in health indicators, thus affecting targets of IMR-MMR
3. Increase in post-surgery
4. Increase in accidents rate
5. Increase the cost of health care delivery.

Reasons for shortage of nurses recruitment and retention, compensation not provided, no benefits so they shift jobs, nurses are qualified, experienced and competent security is not compromised in light if global uncertainty. Code of conducts is internationally recognized, budgetary support. Today less people enter in this profession due to multiple other careers options and better payments and facilities offered in the market. Today good customer service is in demand, patient is better informed. To know even one life has breathed easier because nurses have lived. Nurses are special people tireless hours of care to the suffering rendered by her.

It is legally obligatory that all hospitals must attend emergency patients in the best possible manner. Even if the patient is outside the doctors area of expertise, appropriate first aid must be given and thereafter the patient must be transferred to the appropriate facility. All medical help must be given and then the patient must be transferred to the appropriate facility as soon as possible.

Suggested Precautions

1. *Mixing of patient report*—a potential area of concern, the consequences of which can at times be serious. Cultivating the habit of

reading the names of the patients name on each report before perusing any report or document can minimize this error. On getting the investigation reports specifically note the date and time on which the report is perused in the patient's medical records. The result of each and every investigation report must be briefly written in the prescription slip, case papers. Normal repots write as normal.

2. *Parting with original medical records*—a definite recipe for disaster. Copies of all medical records must be prepared and retained before parting with the originals. Proper endorsement must be taken from the authority seeking possession of the medical record. During reference, transfer, discharge, the patient must be provided the photocopies of the medical reports and not the original records. Investigation reports, X-ray plate have to be handed over to the patient after proper acknowledgement taken as received. Assure care not cure.

3. *Precautions in treating self-medicating patients.* There are some drugs which are relatively contraindicated with others and in case the patient has not disclosed to the doctor about having taken a particular drug and coincidently the contraindicated drug is prescribed, it can and has led to catastrophic consequences hence more care is needed. It is equally important to ensure that the consultants are also available when required and do give advise and in appropriate cases do visit the patient even at odd hours, if the need arises. Any abnormality reported in investigation reports must be taken seriously and suitable steps must be taken. Common advice "take rest" should be given in written. History of patient must not openly be referred, but relevant parts must also be recorded.

4. *Failure to attend an emergency patient*— consumer court directs the doctor to pay compensation. It is legally obligatory that all doctors/hospitals must attend emergency patients in best possible manner. Even if the patient is outside the doctors area of expertise, appropriate first aid must be given and thereafter the patient to be transferred to appropriate facility.

5. *Maintenance and service records of machineries and equipment*—relevance and importance in a court. Always procure a reputed/standard brand and that too from an equally reputed reseller. Preserve the invoice the accompanying literature and other instructions send by the manufacture must be the duly preserved. Nowadays operation instructions or precautions on a CD or on the internet made available, in both cases the print out relevant instructions must be preserved. The instructions for using the machines must be made known to all those who are supposed to operate it or assist in operating it. If the manufacturer offers training then all those who have to handle the machine regular, maintenance and serving followed must attend the same. Operating machine and equipment by unqualified and untrained staff are negligence.

6. *Pathways and lifts to ICU/OT* and operational are always kept clear and and operational in emergency, delay of a few minutes can be considered as negligence. ET tube must be thoroughly checked before inserting, and checked at regular intervals; slipping due to loose tape and kicking are two areas of concern. Failure to foresee an emergency and remaining unprepared to deal with the same could be negligence. Preserve entire medical records of the patient for a period of 3 years. Complete medical records must be produced before the court.

Nurses know this—no neglecting medical negligence: Medical negligence is any case when a health provider deviates from standard care in treating a patient. What to do when you suspect medical negligence:

1. File a complaints with local police, state medical council and state consumer forum

2. Police will send complaint to medical council

3. If medical council upholds complaint, depending on charges made against the doctor/hospital, they will file a case under relevant sections. Case goes to the appropriate court

4. If it is a criminal case, it becomes a case of state versus the doctor/hospital

5. State medical council can initiate action against the doctor by suspending his license to practice for specific period of time or removing his name from medical register depending on seriousness of charges.

6. If charges are upheld in court, doctor can be arrested and jailed

7. If either party is aggrieved by the state medical councils decision, she/he can appeal before the medical council of India.

8. The complainant can take the state medical council decision and approach the consumer court for compensation.

9. If complaint goes to the consumer forum either a panel of medical experts will look into its merits or the forum will send it to the state medical council to do the same.

10. If complaints is upheld forum decides quantum of compensation to be paid to the complainant.

11. Consumer forum can only decide compensation amount but cannot punish anyone even if negligence is proved.

12. If unhappy with the consumer forums decision, any of the parties can appeal before the national consumer disputes redresses commission and further on to supreme court if needed

13. You can also consult patient advocacy groups or legal experts, to help define case and check facts.

14. Keep original records, all diagnosis, procedure, advice is noted down in the prescription file. Do not give originals to anyone.

15. Delhi Medical Council, one of the authorities patients in Delhi and NCR can complain to, gets 20–30 complaints of medical negligence monthly.

New Researches in Surgery

Could replace antibiotics in surgery?
Loading wounds with carbon dioxide gas during surgery could protect the site from air borne bacteria and suffocate germs, according to a study laboratory tests by researchers showed that humidified carbon dioxide would also keep the wound warm and moist, which should reduce tissue damage and speed up healing. The scientist is now planning clinical trials on humans.

New surgery technique makes artificial arms easier to control, allowing them to point a finger, grasp a cricket bat or even give someone a pinch. The technique involves reconnecting amputated nerve fibers to muscles in the chest and using electrical impulses from those nerves to operate a special motorized artificial arm.

Currently most prosthetic arms are powered by body motion. Motion in the upper shoulder is transferred through a cable to operate the hand, wrist or elbow. Nevertheless, this method only allows people to use one joint at a time and takes a lot of training.

Restoring nerve function offers a much more natural way to control the devices and allows people to remove more than one joint at once. The re-attached nerves can be used with a next generation type of prosthetic device to perform complex elbow, wrist and hand movements, better mimicking the function of the lost limb.

The prosthetic devices have antennas that capture electrical impulses from the nerves. These signals are processed by a computer, which directs the arm to perform needed motion.

Now a patient can think I want to close my hands this way with this complex hand, he will be able to do it. With increasing functional capabilities, patients with upper extremity amputations may derive exceptional benefits from prosthetic arms, just as legions of patients with lower extremity amputations no lead remarkably normal and even athletic lives.

Micro camera transforms endoscope surgery—German scientists have invented a low-cost camera that is smaller than a grain of salt but offers razor sharp pictures. Using it, researchers plan to create tiny disposable endoscopes for minimally invasive operations in future disposable endoscopes for minimally invasive operation. A new low cost micro camera is what makes it possible. Digital camera systems consist of two components, a lens and a sensor that transforms the image into electrical signal. Electrical contacts on the sensor allow access to these signals and therefore also the image. Due to the way they are manufactured, these contacts are located between the sensor and the lens.

Scientists grow bones from fat in lab-tech will pave way for repairing or replacing broken bones with new ones. Growing human bones from stem cells. There is a need for artificial bones for injuries and in operation. We use 3 dimensional structures to fabricate the bone in the right shape and geometric. We can grow these bones outside the body and then transplant it to the patient at the right time. By scanning the damaged bone area, the implant should fit perfectly and merge with the surrounding tissue. There are no problems with rejection as the cells come from the patients own body. The scientists were able to insert almost an inch of lab grown human born into the middle section of the rats leg bone. The technique should ultimately allow doctors to replace bones that have been smashed in accidents, fill in defects where bone is missing or carry out reconstruction plastic surgery.

Stem cells give blocked leg veins new life. Adult stem cells extracted from ones own bone marrow have now lent themselves to saving the limbs of people. Vascular surgery—

uses cells to trigger growth of new blood vessel in the limbs of patient suffering from limb ischemia—a condition of blood vessels in the limb getting blocked often resulting in amputation. Patient can walk without pain. Remove the blood from born marrow where high concentrated of stem cells collected. After an angiogram, doctors injected the stem cells into the sport between knee and foot. These sports were along the blocked arteries.

First public bank for cells opens in Chennai, which would store stem cells extracted from a newborns umbilical cord for common use. Stem cells can be send to treat different serious disorders parents can store cord blood for 21 years.

Capsule endoscopies—each capsule contains individual camera which can get in defecation, cost is ₹ 25.000. It helps to study small intestine, upper gastroscopy, lower sigmoidoscopy, small intestine 21 foot long capsules endoscopies takes 8 hours patient swallow and the images are captured on box that is attached to abdomen out side. 8 hours patient come with the box and the readings are taken. There is a magnet that can push the capsule up and down too.

Scientist have developed an intelligent knife that can tell surgeons immediately whether the tissue they are cutting is cancerous or not. The knife is based on electro-surgery, an electrical current rapidly heat tissue, cutting through it while minimizing blood loss. In doing so, they vaporize the tissue, creating smoke that is sucked by extraction systems. This smoke would be a rich source of biological information, he connected an electrosurgical knife to a mass spectrometer, an analytical instrument used to identify what chemicals are present in a sample, different types of cell produce 1000 of metabolites in different concentrations, so the profile of chemicals in a biological sample can reveal information about the state of that tissue. The knife works by matching its readings during surgery to the reference library to determine what type of tissue is being cut, giving a result in less than 3 seconds. The technology was then transferred to the OT to perform real time analysis during surgery tests matched postoperation diagnosis biased on traditional methods. Current study focused on cancer diagnosis, it can also identify many other features, such as tissue with an inadequate blood supply or types bacteria present in the tissues.

LASER THERAPY

Laser (light amplification by stimulated emission of radiation) is being used increasingly for scientific, industrial and military purposes. Laser acts as a precision blood vessels, light scalpel or can be used for photocoagulation.

Types

1. Carbon dioxide laser is the most commonly used laser for otohinolaryngology and general surgery. It results in immediate tissue destructions precise and clean surgery, minimal damage to surrounding tissues, bloodless dissection by sealing the small blood vessels, healing in a rapid manner. It can be used free hand or through a surgical binocular microscope.
2. Argon laser produces photocoagulation of reefing and blood vessels. It has been utilized for stapedectomy, middle ear surgery and hemahgiomas.
3. Nd:YAG laser has been recently introduced and produces slow adequate tissue destruction with minimum bleeding. It is also being tried for destroying opaque lesions in the eye, and calculi in kidneys and gall bladder. It is used for endo-bronchial surgery.

Effects

- *Thermal:* It produces vaporization of water in cells by heating.
- *Non-thermal:* Photomechanical and photochemical changes occur. It is being

tried for destruction of renal and gall stones.
- Biostimulation may occur at low does.

Indications

Microlaryngeal surgery can be performed by carbon dioxide laser. It can be used for treatment of vocal nodules, polyps, laryngeal stenosis, papillotten bilateral vocal cord palsy and malignancy.

Oral cavity: Benig and malignant lesions may be excised.

Pharyngeal pouch may be treated endo-scopically by laser.

Endoscopic surgery of bronchial free and esophagus can be performed by laser therapy.

Otology: Nyringotomy and stapedectomy are being tried by laser. Acoustic neuromata also have been excised by laser.

Nose Rhinophyma, polyps, adhesions, etc. have been treated by laser surgery. Palliative treatment for advanced malignancy is possible.

Technique: Carbon dioxide laser is the most commonly used. It is delivered by connecting it to the binocular operating microscope under GA patient with complete muscular relaxation when laser is being used. Duration of laser surgery for each area is less then one second.

Complications

- Eyes can be damaged by its exposure. The patient and personnel in OT must wear goggles to prevent direct or reflected exposure to laser.
- Anesthetic tube must be protected by metal foils or it should be made of flexible metallic tube to prevent damage of the tube by laser, which may result in explosion.
- Skin may be burnt by exposure.
- Vocal cord may be damaged.
- Tracheal perforation is possible while performing laser bronchoscopy.

Advantages

Precision surgery is possible minimum bleeding is a great advantage minimum tissue reaction occurs.

Disadvantages

Cost of laser therapy is very high; biopsy may not be possible as the tissue is excised by destruction. Trauma may occur to the patient and the patient and personnel in the OT.

Cryosurgery

Cryosurgery utilizes freezing for excision of tissues with the help of cryoprobe.

Mode of Action

- The living tissues get destroyed, if it is frozen by applying a very cold probe. Majority of living tissues die on freezing to temperature below –20°C for longer than a minute. This can happen in many ways.
- Cell membrane ruptures due to the formation of ultracellular ice crystals.
- Intracellular dehydration occurs due to ice crystallization.
- Protein become denatured.
- Enzymatic inhibition follows destruction of all cellular metabolisms.
- Local ischemia and microthrombosis of blood vessels occur.

Clinical Progress

- Freezing of the tissues occurs.
- Normal appearance of the tissue is regained after cryosurgery as the ice crystals throw out.
- Inflammation soon follows with hyperemia.
- Necrosis sets in with slough formation.
- Healthy granulations cover the tissues when the slough separates.
- Rapid healing occurs with the formation of new epithelium with minimum scanning or distortion.

Degree of Cryonecrosis

Depends on temperature of the probe, size of the probe duration of cryotherapy number of applications, vascularity of the area, density of the tissue.

Indication

1. *Oncology:* Malignant tumors are treated palliatively by cryosurgery. It produces relief from pain and the tumors can regress. Since the bones are not destroyed by freezing maligned tissues can be destroyed without producing any necrosis. Localized destruction can be obtained with minimum bleeding under local (CA) or sedation. The procedure can be performed repeatedly. Tumors of oral cavity and phazynx can be controlled by cryopobe, benign tumors like pupilomata hemangioma, angiofibroma and glomus can be treated.
2. *Oral cavity*
   - Tonsillectomy is performed for patients with bleeding dyscrasias or when GA is contraindicated. It can be used to destroy tonsilar remnants.
   - Granular pharyngitis can be treated.
   - Ulcers like aphthous and hepatic ulcers may respond to cryotherapy.
   - Epulis can be treated by freezing.
3. *Nasal cavity:* Epistaxis may be controlled by freezing but recurrence may occur. Vasomotor rhinitis hypertrophic turbinates nasal polyps may be treated by the therapy.
4. *Ear:* Menjere's disease may respond therapy. Bleeding is minimum, pain is negligible.

Disadvantages

Efficacy is often limited.

Histopathology of the excised tissue is not possible due to destruction of the tissue by freezing. Physiology is an ever-changing field.

Preparing a sterile field using a commercially prepared sterile kit/tray—a sterile field is created to provide a surgically aseptic workplace. It should be considered a restricted area. Commercially prepared sterile kits and trays are wrapped that, once opened, becomes the sterile field. If the area is breached, the entire sterile field is considered contaminated. A sterile field is created to provide a surgically aseptic workplace. It should be considered a restricted area. The sterile drape should be waterproof on one side, with that side placed down on the work surface.

Spider Tech

1. *What is spider tech?* Surgeons in Delhi will for the first time in Asia pacific used a pioneering technology called "spider technology", a single flexible laparoscopy instrument that will do away with the need for five incisions or scars for any abdominal intervention. Instead, the rod like machine will enter through the belly but ton and open up like an umbrella within the abdomen, providing the surgeon with several instruments with 300° range of motion along with small cameras. Once the procedure is completed, the system closes up and is removed through the same incision.

2. *Where is it done in India?* It was first done for the first time by doctor Pradeep Chowdery, who heads the Max institute of minimal access. Metabolic and Bar iatric surgery in Delhi. It also happens to be the first operation in Asia Pacific. The surgery was conducted on July 10th 2012.

3. *Why earlier technology was painful?* Earlier for any abdominal surgery doctors made 3–4 extrapunctures for different instruments to go in, leaving multiple scars 5–10 mm in diameter. Over all the process was painful which left deep scars on the body.

4. *Where will spider tech come handy?* This scar less rout will be used to treat common abdominal conditions like appendix, gall bladder stones and the weight loss barbaric surgeries. This is a quantum jump from the rigid laparoscopy. Greatest benefit is that there will be no visible scar because the spider enters the abdomen through a small puncture at the naval or umbilicus hence resulting in virtually a scar less surgery with excellent cosmetic outcomes.

5. *How does it function?* The spider is a flexible operating platform, which has multiple arms, each acting as a separate instrument. The instrument will go in and open up like an umbrella. The different limbs have different function. One could be a holder, a dissector and the other a clip applier. Patients who receive a spider surgical procedure may experience less scarring with the potential for limited postoperative pain. A water proof dressing is done on the belly button after the instrument is taken out and there will be no stitches.

6. *Which country is it done?* India, UK, USA, China, South Africa, Germany, Australia, Japan, Canada, France.

7. *What is the price?* According to the doctor, getting operated with a spider technology will cost around 30.000 more than a normal laparoscopy surgery. In India it will amount to nearly 60.000.

Medical Revolution

Nursing education has moved, re-looked at as changing role of a nurse—it is a need of the hour.

- We live in a world that is constantly growing smaller and our planet shrinking. Scientific technology in medical field spreading faster than ever before
- Nursing is an applied science, the better the scientific background the safer and more intelligent will be the care the nurse renders.
- The increasing competitiveness in the work culture today, with new age race, eagerness to excel, constant up date and keep up with new trends that are changing like world wind

Modern computer: Today the man has come a long way now, you would hardly find an area of modern living that is not yet touched by the computer. Telecommunication, defense preparedness, medical and space research, railway booking, electricity billing, on line shopping, the computer controls most of the activities. Computer science is now being offered as a core subject in schools and colleges.

Superior computers are the largest, fastest and most expensive computers made so far which has memory of 256 megabytes, e.g. it operates at speeds of 1.2 billion flops. It can perform calculations in minute, which a personal computer could perform in three weeks.

Buggy computer researchers have discovered that the structural arrangement futuristic computes that use light rather than electricity to process information.

Computer system comes with several communication devices that all know, that you can use to communicate over internet, some devices come in built and others are attached to your computer. Telephone lines, speakers, headphones, mike, digital camera, MP3 players an many other accessories, it also connected electronic mail, online banking, travel, fax machine, web camera/video camera where current images can be had from a website. A live camera is one that is continually providing new images that are transmitted in rapid succession. Microsoft have revolutionaries the working experience on personal computer with its wide range of operating system and office automation applications due to the interactive user, interface and simplicity of use, it has gained popularity. It has unlimited storage capacity, an small pen drive can store entire institutional data and it can be made available for verification when as and when we need.

Highly Technical

Medicines moved from the organism to organ and from organ to cells to molecular properties manipulation of body and mind, that is genetic counseling. Genetic engineering, parental diagnosis of sex, in vitro fertilization, storing eggs (technology allows freezing and storing of healthy eggs to be used later). Embryo adoption (it is a relatively newer method and steadily gaining ground. Couples are adopting an embryo rather than a child. It works in combination with infertility technique) cloning, organ transplantation. The use of artificial kidney machine, Stem cells, Teddy robot to help with patient care and Robots with ethics. Micro camera transforms endoscope surgery, Scientists grow bones from fat in lab cosmetic surgery. Injecting oxygen into blood could help keep people alive, the list is very long.

We are living in an unparalleled time for technological progress. In 10 years, it will be almost impossible to describe to any child in India, what life was like before the internet.

About 2 billion of the world's 7 billion people have an internet connections and remaining 5 billion will get one in next decade. Almost one billion of them will come on line in India.

Knowledge can be disseminated more widely than ever. The internet has connected great teachers to villages across remote parts of India.

With advance of the internet, the newest modality of learning in information technology we can continue medical education at website. Only one has to have internet and access to right kind of information—there you find visuals, research reports, and learn about your topic as you search. Today nurse is not merely attendant in the ill room but also an educator and researcher, which will help her to come up the level of accuracy and will be able to respond to the challenges. We have to walk those extra miles. Motivation is the power that drives a person from within to act, if you have will to go beyond the ordinary, there are tools to take you there.

There fore re-write your destiny people with drive and ambitions the world is truly not enough. Our mind is like soft sponge that can absorb maximum, man is truly an amazing being. He is master of inventors. He is restless by nature, he dives his imagination to keep inventing. We live in age of technology; every nurse is required to keep herself aware of digital gadgets.

Medical subjects are giant, one can never dive into its depth, and one has to keep informed ourselves everyday, even at my age I feel a drop in the ocean in spite of extensive reading. We have a wider role to become a new age nurses with today's rapid and unprecedented changes there is an new urgency of knowledge that is indispensable to deal with multidimensional situation. Knowledge is power, an asset and greatest weapon of our lives/times. Real knowledge is highest value and not obtained easily, to get you have to struggle.

You know that today—sophisticated technology can prolong life well beyond the time when death would have occurred in the past, e.g. earlier days when a doctor could do nothing more for a critically ill person, the family would start praying, now they turn to the internet which provides wealth of information.

There was a time not so long ago when getting a second opinion was difficult. Today remote diagnosis is possible.

Expensive experimental procedures and medications are available, harvesting and freezing of life, premature infants are given a chance to survive with technical support, and today life expectancy has increased with better quality of life possible.

Such expanded level mean, patient empowerment and more democratization.

Computerization in medical field has helped to improve efficiency at work, improve the services, provide better professional care and improve profitability. It is a powerful tool. Doors are open, only you have to enter in:

- *The mind is tool* change the state of your mind, move forward in new prosperous directions. There is an endless inexhaustible supply of resources and power within you. An ocean of abundance waiting with open hands with un-limited choices, change can begin in this movement. Our minds create our future.
- Our current thinking shapes the future.
- The action of today becomes the destiny of tomorrow
- If a child gave up at the first fall, he would never learn to walk. Do not be in hurry, as you cannot travel a long journey in a single day. The process of learning is always same; you are not perfect the first day.
- Tagor "a lamp can never light another lamp unless it burns on its own wick" teachers are essential knowledge builders, torch-bearers. It is said that a good teacher explains, a superior teacher demonstrates and an exceptional teacher inspires, she is a maker of man, she can mould the minds with sound knowledge, where students can drink from running stream. Without a good teacher the best system of education is bound to fall and with good teachers defects of system can overcome.

Stress among Nursing Professionals

- Currently major concern—overburden, underemployment and underpayment along with own personal reasons. Work load, shift work, lack of reward (not paid to the proportion to their quality and no incentive for good performance) work place stress, hectic time schedule, leadership style, professional conflicts, traveling, social and family stress, increased expectations and desires, unnecessary worries all these reads to a burn out and rise the symptoms of irritation, short temper, anxiety, inability to concentrate, negative attitude, emotional exhaustion, decreased personal accomplishments and physiological symptoms and diseases.

Secrets of success are to aim high, be cool, every minute is precious, be uptodate, push hard to achieve your goal. Be strong enough to face the world each day. Be weak enough to know you cannot do everything. Be generous to those who need your help. Be the first to congratulate an opponent who succeeds. Be yourself always. The road to success is not straight, there is a curve called failure, a loop called confusion, red light called enemies and caution light called family. Nevertheless, if you have an engine called perseverance, insurance called faith, a guide called Jesus; you will make it to a place called success.

Chapter 29

Burn Wound Management (Medically and Surgically)

Burns Patient in Emergency Service

1. Receive patient in ER room
2. Get details from relatives, initiate outpatient, and inpatient record.
3. Contact specialist
4. Immediately start IV line with IV cannula 18, if not possible with 20. CVP line if necessary.
5. Simultaneously take blood for CBC, blood group, renal panel and electrolytes
6. Record vital signs
7. Fluid first 24 hours ringer lactate solution; if major burns first little to be given in 1–2 hours.
8. Nil oral if major burns
9. Catheterization and start input outputs chart
10. Start oxygen by mask
11. Wound swab taken local application of silver sulphadiazine, after aspiration of blister, blisters should not be opened
12. Blood samples sent for preanesthetic panel and help panel
13. Inform emergency room doctor as soon as patient is brought
14. Doctor will give analgesia. For major burns given injection Fortwin 15 mg and injection Phenergan 25 mg I/M if patient is more than 50 kg weight
15. Injection glycopyuvate 1 cc IM
16. Give injection tetanus toxoid
17. If electrical burns, cardiology opinion is taken
18. When inhalation burns are suspected, ABG to be done and pulmonology opinion is taken
19. When burn to eyes present ophthalmology consultation is obtained
20. Foley catheter put in and retained
21. Assess the degree of burn by rule of nine
22. Consult the plastic surgeon
23. Start antibiotics
24. Intravenous access—peripheral/central line inserted
25. Calculate fluid to be replaced in the 1st 24 hours by Parkland formula
26. Arrange for an AC room and specialized nursing care
27. Inform the relatives about the seriousness of burns, prognosis and financial concerns
28. Rehydration started following the parklands formula

Local Management of Burns

Level of ICU care

1. Level-1—provides monitoring, observation and short term ventilation
2. Level-2—provides observation, monitoring and long term ventilation with resident doctors
3. Level-3—provides all aspects of intensive care including invasive hemodynamic monitoring and dialysis.

Bed Space and Beds

a. All separate cubic
b. 225–250 square feet per beds
c. Beds-adjustable, no head board, side rails and with wheels, remote controlled with faculty for all positioning for nursing care and physiotherapy and emergency situations.

Lighting

1. Light should be adequate for routine nursing task yet a soft luminous lighting
2. Total luminosity should not exceed 30 foot candle
3. Maximum night lighting should not exceed 6.5 foot candle.

Dressing Techniques

a. Open *vs* closed
b. Ointment *vs* cream
c. Daily or alternate day
d. Anesthesia or analgesia
e. Early excision *vs* delayed excision
f. Meshed grafts *vs* Meek micrografting *vs* sheet graft
g. Anchoring sutures *vs* Staples

1. *Primary treatment:* All blisters and devitalized tissues to be removed radically and kollagen-M applied. 48 hours later wound check. Kollagen-M well stuck can be left alone covered or uncovered until it starts falling off. Superficial burns healing completed under kollagen. Deep burns need to be grafted.
2. *Kollages:* Uses form a protective barrier between body and atmosphere which will prevents entry of bacteria. Prevents excessive loss of plasma, decrease pain, decrease frequency of dressing.
3. *Open vs closed:* All burn wounds to be kept covered. Face wounds are the only wounds, which can be kept open. Closed technique prevents friction between wound and bed clothes, prevents gross

infection by allowing ointment or cream to remain in touch with the wound all through without getting wiped off, decreases pain by covering the exposed raw areas.

4. *Ointment vs cream:* Initially sliver sulphadiazine cream till slough comes out. Later Betadine ointment. Mupirocin cream—if MRSA positive. If wound too wet—Betadine ointment even if slough not yet come out.
5. Daily dressing is must if discharge is copious if SSD used. Alternate day dressing good enough when discharge is not significant and povidone iodine is used. Sometimes even twice a day dressing are done in case of copious discharge.
6. No anesthesia, analgesia round the clock and stepped up before and during the dressing. A combination of tramadol, ketamine and midazolam
7. Always early excision if patient comes early enough and facilities exist. Early enough is up to 72 hours post burn. Early excision decreases the chances of sepsis and facilitates early mobilization and better and more predictable functional recovery. Delayed excision is generally at 3 weeks or later.
8. Dermatome-harvesting graft, meshed skin grafts are done in skin grafting
9. Acute burns always meshed or meek micrografting for better takes. Reconstructive procedures like over grafting and release of contractures always sheet grafting for better cosmesis. Meek micrografting gives wider coverage and more predictable takes than mesh grafting but more expensive.
10. Positioning on plate, adhesive spraying, dermatome cut through, cork removing, gauze expansion, micrograft positioning, after gauze removal 7th day, 10th day wound care given.
11. These days the skin grafts are encored with surgical staples and not sutures as

the procedure is faster saves anesthesia time and lesser chances of infection.

12. Areas easy and quick to excise—trunk and legs, joints and throats, hands and face

13. *Allograft:* Classic benefits in water, electrolyte and protein loss. Reduction in energy requirements secondary to the attainment of a closed wound. Reduction in wound infection rates, reduction in pain, conservation of autograft, improved general welfare and psychological outlook of the patient.

14. *Alloderm:* Processed human cadaveric skin, removed epidermis, extracted dermal cells, template for dermal regeneration, good take rates, reduce subsequent scarring, allowing grafting of an ultrathin spilt skin graft a one stage procedure.

15. Integra is most widely accepted synthetic skin substitute, Bilaminar structure, the median take is 85%, two-stage procedure, with a minimum interval of 3 weeks between the application of the Integra and the spilt skin grafting. It is relatively expensive.

16. Grown in vitro and then applied to wounds. Take of cultures epithelial auto-grafts depends on the wound bed. Expensive, skilled labour and quality control, 3–5 weeks to produce, fragile sheets, blistering, infection, and contractures.

Burn Wound Management

1. At risk groups deep circumferential limb or truncal burns, high voltage electrical injuries, delayed resuscitation.

2. Signs and symptoms—cyanosis of distal un-burnt limb skin, unrelenting deep pain, progressive parenthesis, progressive decrease, absence of pulse.

3. Edema under escheat, remove all rings, jewelry, elevate, active motion, check skin color, sensation, capillary refill, Doppler pulses.

Principles of Wound Management

1. *Control or eliminate a causative factor that is pressure:* (assessment of skin, change of position, prevention of moisture, pressure relieving mattresses, and compression devices), *shear, friction* (use of turn sheet or trapeze while moving the patient, using heel protectors, a knee catch in propped up position, light dusting of powder or corn starch on sheets to reduce friction), moisture (from continuous incontinence or sweating such as bowel/bladder training, external collecting devices and meticulous skin care) *and circulatory impairment and neuropathy* (measure to promote blood flow to ischemic areas such as hydration, eliminating of nicotine and caffeine and avoidance of cold environment, compression devices for prevention of DVT, glycemic control for prevention of neuropathy).

2. *Provide systemic support* for healing through nutritional and fluid support, promotion of tissue oxygenation and control of factors deterrent to wound healing (assessment of body weight, serum albumin, prealbumin and transferring levels, current total oral intake of calories and proteins, clinical indicators of malnutrition such as joint edema, dry skin, provision of oral, entral and parenteral support and provision of vitamin and mineral supplements, promotion of tissue oxygenation—hydration, elevation, administration of oxygenation, vigilance in vital check and control of factors deterrent to wound healing)

3. *Maintain physiologic local wound environment* prevent and manage infection, cleanse wound, remove non-viable tissue, maintain appropriate level of moisture, eliminate dead space, control odor, eliminate pain and protect per wound skin (promote adequate moisture level, temperature control, PH regulation, local blood supply and control of bacterial burden.

Prevent and Manage Infection

a. By appropriate wound dressing, impermeable to bacteria, based on the wound assessment, infection control precautions, appropriate wound cleansing and debridement, antimicrobials if needed.

b. Cleaning wound NS with 4–15 PSI (pound per square inch) of pressure to remove debris without harming healthy tissue.

c. Remove non viable tissues by appropriate debridement methods, select topical dressings that maintain moist environment to prevent tissue desiccation.

d. Maintain appropriate level of moisture

e. Eliminate dead space

f. Control odor

g. Minimize pain

h. Proper interval to wound change

Types of dressing: Hydrocolloid dressing; hydrogel dressings, alginate dressing, semipermeable film dressings, deodorizing dressings, iodine dressings, silver dressings, low-non-adherent and membrane dressings, honey dressings, other dressings.

Infection control measures: Use of sterile dressings, use of sterile cotton tipped applicators for inserting wound fillers, gauze or packaging material, irritants solutions and devices used to hold the solution as well as administer the irritants should be sterile. Surface of dressing that will touch the wound should not be touched with any un-sterile article. Standard precautions should be followed.

Dressing removal is done on a scheduled basis depending upon the type of dressing; dressing that are over saturated or leaking should be changed immediately. Adhesive should be removed can be used to moisten the dressing if it is attached to the wound base. Gently roll or lift an edge of the dressing to get a starting edge. Support the tissue adjacent to the dressing.

Wound cleanings: NS is an effective cleansing agent when delivered to the wound site with adequate force to agitate and wash away the surface debris and devitalized tissue that may harbors bacteria.

Dressing application: After dressing removal and wound cleansing the surrounding skin is gently cleansed and dried. Skin scalant may be applied to the skin before applying the dressing to protect the skin. Then, apply the selected dressing according to the instruction without stretching the skin. In glutei folds, wafer dressings are folded in half before application to ensure that the adhesive seals into the anatomic contours. Application of dressing to the heel or elbow requires cutting and shaping the dressing to customize the fit.

Wound packing and filling: If tunneling is present strip gauze packing is used to fill narrow areas, allow for dressing retrieval. For large, deep wounds, hydrating or absorbent-impregnated gauze is effective. Packing material should be fluffed and loosely placed into the wound with edges and bases. Gauze dressing is applied as an additional absorbent layer and a secondary cover dressing is applied and secured.

Selecting the dressing: Self-adhesive wraps, tape, Montgomery straps or gauze wraps may be used for securing the dressing.

Education: For patient's knowledge and understanding are major factor in compliance with treatment regimes. Verbal education should be reinforced by written information.

Types of wound: Laceration, incision, abrasion, contusion and puncture wound.

Bleeding: According to the blood vessel involves arterial, venous and capillary type

Site of bleeding is internal and external.

Tissue type wound bed: It is necrotic (black), sloughy (yellow) and granulating (red) Epithelializing (pink) and hypergranulating (red) hematoma.

Dimension of wound—length, width, depth in cm/mm or trace wound circumference.

Pathological stage—noninfected and infected

Drainage color serous (straw), haemoserous (red/straw), purulent (green/brown/yellow)

Amount—low, moderate, high

Consistency—clear, hazy

Wound healing, or cicatrisation, is an intricate process

- Homeostasis—after initial wounding, the blood vessels in the wound bed contract and a clot is formed. Within minutes post in-injury, platelets aggregate at the injury site to form a fibrin clot. This clot acts to control active bleeding. This achieves homeostasis.
- Inflammatory—blood vessels dilate to allow essential cells, antibodies, white blood cells, growth factor enzymes and nutrient in the wounded area.
- Proliferate stage—during proliferation, the wound is rebuilt with new granulation tissue, and this will be seen by the end of first week till wound is healed it will continue.
- Remodeling—maturation is the final phase and occurs once the wound is closed. There is a lot of activity still happening after wound has healed on the surface. This final phase continues for up to 18 months after your wound is closed.

Types of Wound Healing

- Primary intension—healing occurs in wound that have minimal tissue loss and when edges are well closed. If there are no complications, such as infection, necrosis, or abnormal scar formation, wound healing occurs with minimal granulation tissue and scarring.
- Secondary intension—healing is seen in wounds with extensive tissue loss and wounds in which the edges can not be closed. The wound is left open, and

granulation tissue gradually fills in the deficit. Repair time is longer, tissue replacement and scarring are greater and the susceptibility to infection is increased due to lack of an epidermal barrier to microorganism.

- Tertiary intension—healing also known as delayed or secondary closing. Suturing of the wound is delayed until the problems resolve and more favorable conditions exist for wound healing.
- Factors affecting wound healing—mechanical, edema, ischemia and necrosis, foreign bodies, low oxygen tension. Inadequate perfusion, inflammation, nutrient, metabolic diseases, immuno-suppressant, connective tissue disorders, smoking.
- Complication of wounds—wound bleeding may indicate a dislodged clot, slipped sutures, coagulation problems, and trauma to blood vessels or tissues, dehiscence, keloid, evisceration, wound infection.
- Wound management—cleaning, closure, dressing and diet.
- Wound cleaning helps optimize the healing environment and decrease the potential for infection. It loosens and washes away cellular debris such as bacteria, purulent material and residual topical agents from previous dressings. NS is preferred cleanser for most wounds because it is physiologic and will always the safe.
- Wound closure maintains a high humidity at the site while removing excess exudates, free of particles and wound contaminants. Non-toxic and can removed without causing trauma to the wound.
- Good nutrition is necessary for healing process, as body needs increased amount of calories, protein, vitamins.
- Wound infection is a serious problem; it results in increased admission to critical care, length of stay, cost of care and death. Osteomyelitis may occur and increases risk of bacteremia, sepsis and multisystem

organ failure. Acute and chronic wounds are booth at risk of infection.

- Contamination is the presence of non-replicating microorganisms on the wound surface.
- Colonization is the presence of replicating bacteria without a host reaction or clinical signs and symptoms of infection.

Acute Wound Infections

a. Surgical site infection occurs within 30 days of surgery and within one year in case of implants. Wound culture is indicated when signs of infection are present or clean wounds does not show any progress in healing in two weeks time. It is taken from healthy tissue as infection involves tissues. It is important to culture rather than pus, slough, echar or necrosis material. The three types of wound culture are wound biopsy, needle aspiration culture and swab culture.
b. Stitch abscess
c. Episiotomy infection
d. Newborn circumcision site infection
e. Infected burns

Role of a nurse in pain management: Pain assessment; record keeping; pre-emptive analgesia administration; explanation and reassurance; distraction and nonpharmacological therapy; dressing technique and dressing choice.

Measures to reduce pain during dressing: Flush, do not rub, when cleansing. Avoid unnecessary stimulus to the wound. Protect wound edges with barrier. Encourage slow, rhythmic breathing and other relaxation techniques. Medicate prior to dressing change and debridement. Avoid aggressive packing.

Mechanism of wound healing—regardless of the type or severity of injury, repair occurs by only two mechanism—regeneration, or replacement of the damaged or lost tissue with more of the same, and scar formation, replacement of damaged or lose tissue by connective tissue that lacks some of the function of the original tissues. Human have only limited capacity for regeneration, and most wounds heal by scar formation. Healing depends on tissue layers involved, onset and duration and type of wound closure.

Wound healing is a series of events. Normally wound healing is initiated by an injury that leads to clot formation and platelet deregulation, is controlled by a myriad of cytokines and growth factors, and is affected significantly by systemic factors such as perfusion, nutritional status and steroid levels.

Wound problems have been present as long as man has been on earth. The cost of treating problem wounds in most industrialized countries is very high.

Wound debridement: The removal of devitalized tissue contaminated by bacteria and foreign bodies, therapy protecting the patient from invasion of bacteria. 3 types debridement—natural, mechanical and surgical.

1. *Natural debridement*—the dead tissue separates from the underlying viable tissue spontaneously.
2. *Mechanical debridement*—involves the use of surgical scissors, scalpels and forceps to separate and remove. This technique can be performed by skilled physician/nurse with daily dressing changes which aid the removal of wound debris. Chemical debridement.
3. *Surgical debridement*—early surgical excision to remove devitalized tissue by operative procedure, ideally, the wound is covered immediately with a skin graft.

Chapter 30

Examples of Surgical Procedures

What is Stents?

Stents are tiny medical devices that are pushed up in the patients block artery. Some stents contains medicine that helps keep the recently unclogged artery open. They are expensive; ₹ 80.000 and have short shelf life of 6 months to 1 year.

Coronary angioplasty is a procedure used to open blocked/clogged arteries of the heart. An angioplasty involves temporary inserting and bowing up a tiny balloon to help widen the artery, cardiologist need at time to place a wire mesh tube like scaffolding used during construction of buildings called a stent to keep the artery from narrowing again. Some stents are coated with medicine to help keep arteries open (drug eluting stents) while others are not baremeta stents)

Two types of stent used in patient such as Bare metal stent; and drug coated stent which has a coating of drug in it. This drug is released in micro concentration after the stent is put in the body. The expiry date for stents varies from 11 months to 2 years.

Part to be operated should be still, 'Dry', Relaxed.

Types of Heart Diseases

- *Congenital:*
  - Acyanotic
  - Cyanotic
  - Valvular

- *Acquired:*
  - RHD
  - IHD
  - Tumors
  - Cardiomyopathies, EMF

Myocardial Blood Supply

- Heart muscle though 'handles' blood cannot use blood for self directly Heart muscle gets its blood supply through separate arteries—coronary arteries. At rest itself, all the oxygen from coronary arterial blood is fully utilized. So, more work = more blood
- *Open heart:* Using heart lung machine, heart is stopped, and operation is performed
- *Close heart:* Operation is performed while heart is beating.

Basic Steps of OHS

- Opening of the chest
- Connect the patient to CPB after heparinisation—'total' CPB
- Cool, stop the heart by cross clamp and cardioplegia
- Open the heart—perform intracardiac operation
- Close cardiotomies—deair the heart
- Declamp, give rest to the heart, wean-off CPB
- Close the chest by keeping the drains

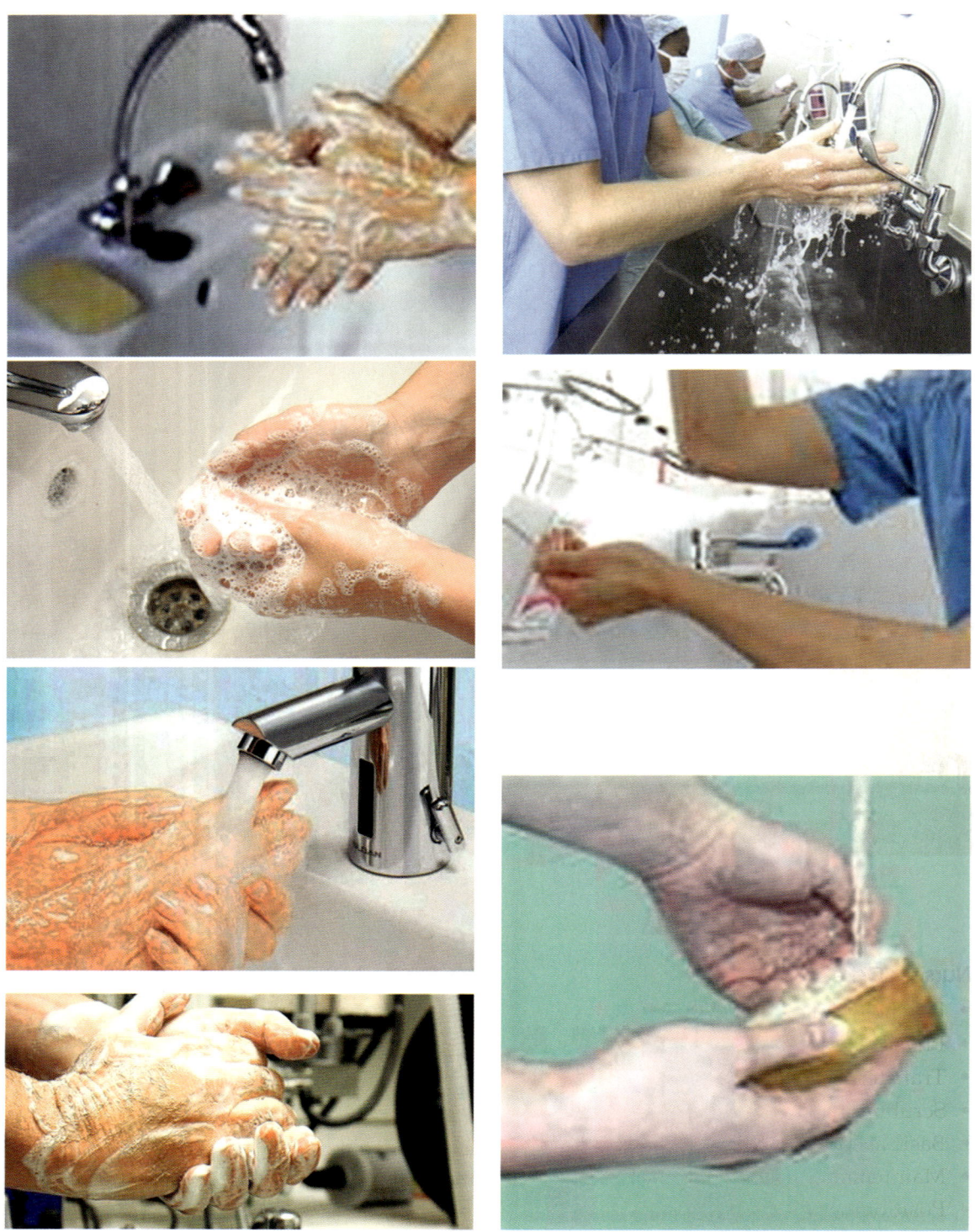

Fig. 30.1: Scrub or surgical handwashing technique procedure

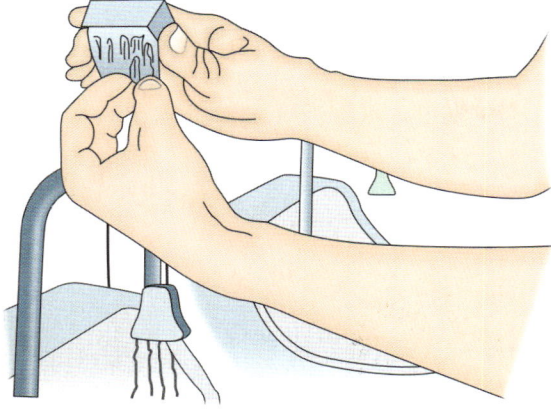
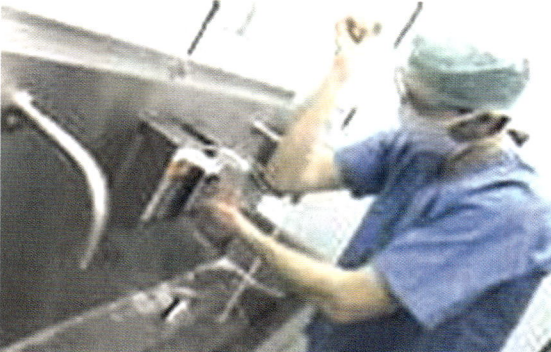
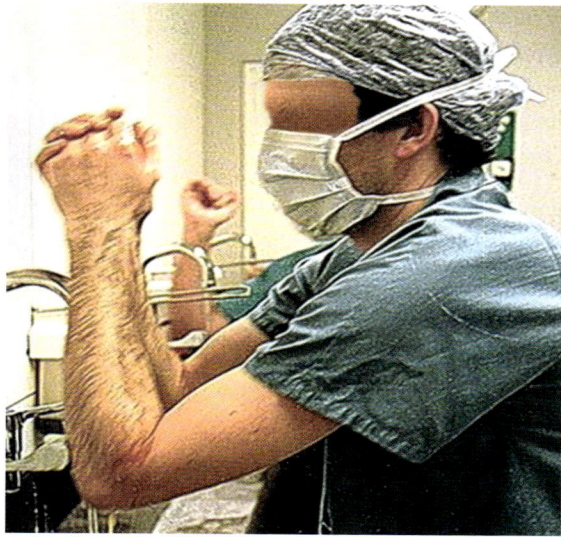
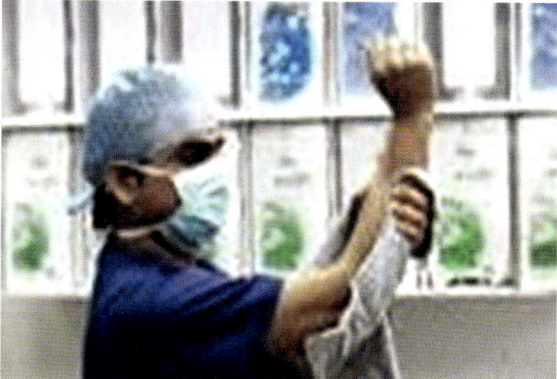

Fig. 30.2: Handwash technique

Nursing Care

- Psychosocial assessment
- Physical assessment
- Transferring the patient
- Scrubbing, gowning and gloving
- Basic aseptic technique
- Maintenance of safety
- Positioning the patient
- Preparing the surgical site
- Patient after surgery

Postoperative Complications

- Myocardial infarction
- Low cardiac output state
- Hemorrhage
- Cardiac tamponade
- Dysrhythmias
- Thrombotic/embolic complications
- Respiratory complications
- Coagulation problems: Renal dysfunction
- Fever/infection
- Altered CNS

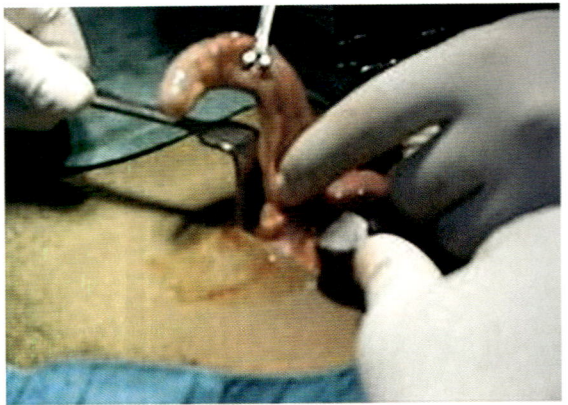

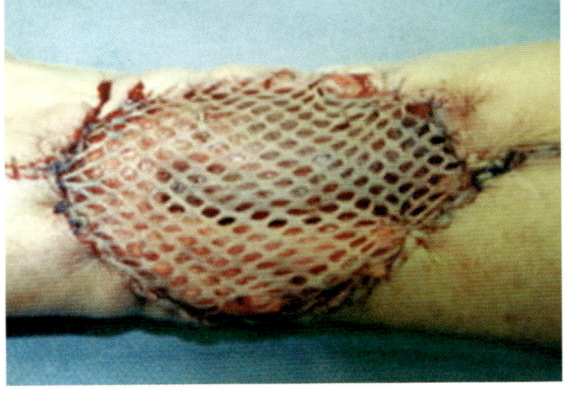

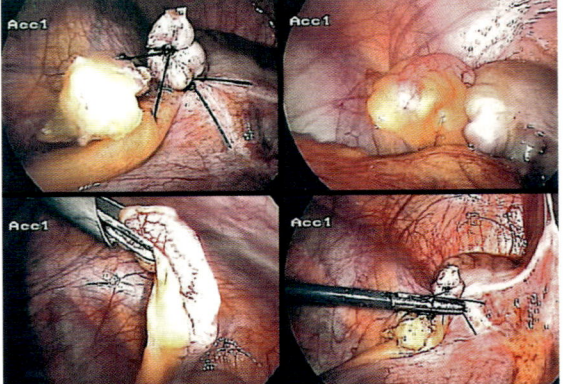

Fig. 30.3: Appendix operation

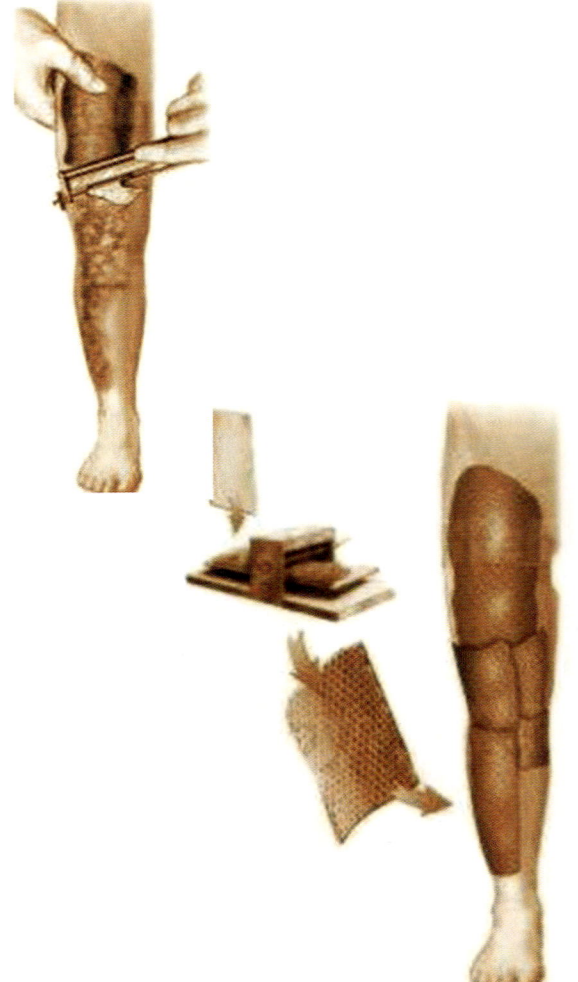

Fig. 30.4: Pancreas surgery (pancreas transplant/islet cell transplant)

Fig. 30.5A: Skin grafting

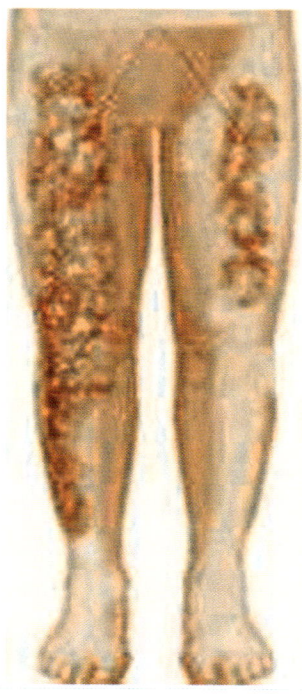

Fig. 30.5B: Skin grafting

New Emerging Procedures

- AF surgery
- Heart failure surgery
- Endovascular surgery
- Minimal access and robotic surgery
- Coronary artery surgery

POLYPECTOMY

Polypectomy is procedure done by doctor under observation of anesthetic by using snare to remove polyp. After the procedure the sample of biopsy is sent.

Banding procedure done to control active bleeding or prevent further complication. It is done for therapeutic purpose. It is known as esophageal vertical ligation.

Procedure

1. Explain the procedure and its charges to client and the relatives
2. Get informed consent
3. Keep client NBM

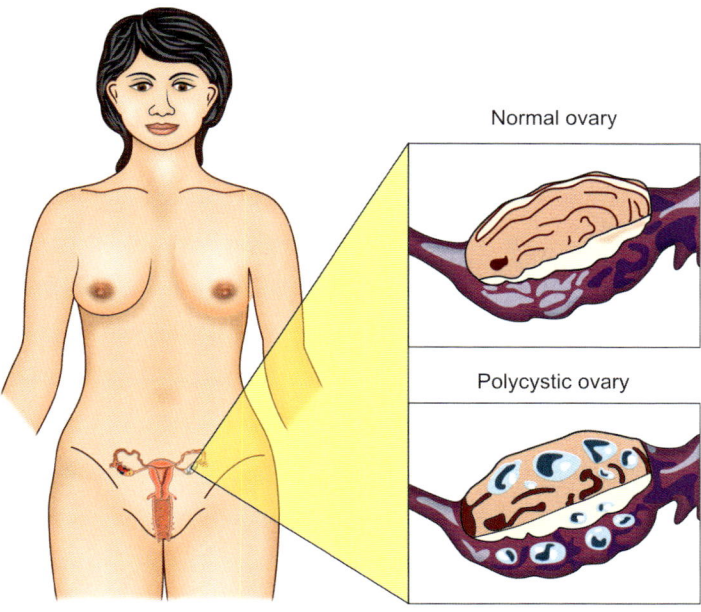

Normal ovary

Polycystic ovary

Fig. 30.6: Polycystic ovary removal

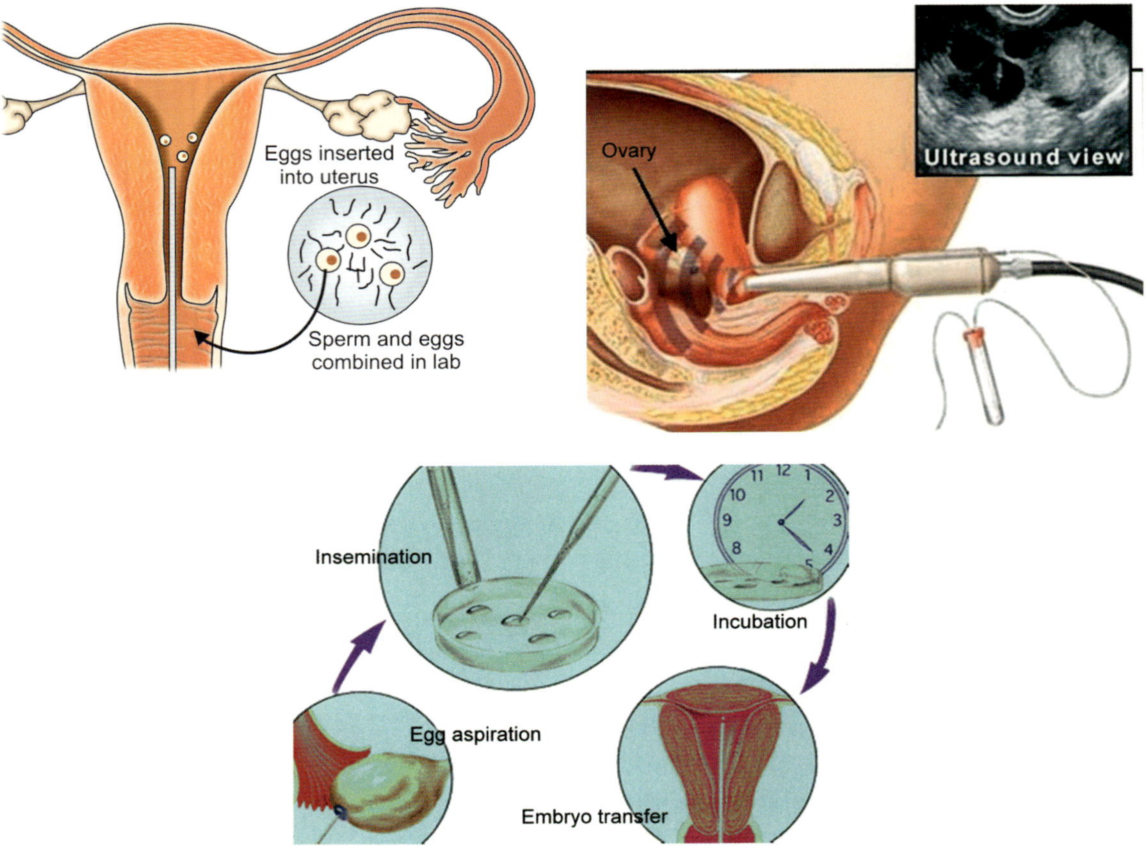

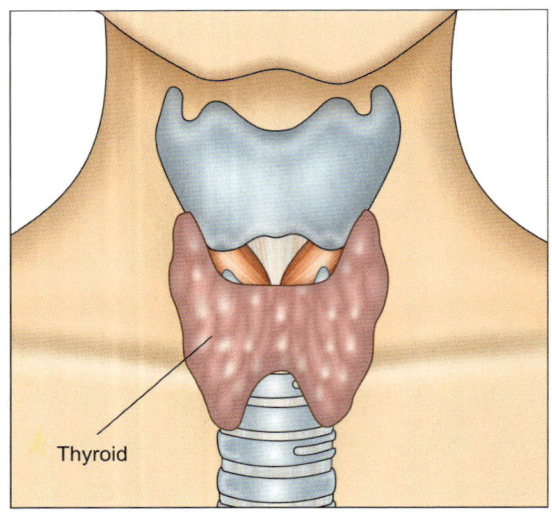

Fig. 30.7: Gynecological procedure

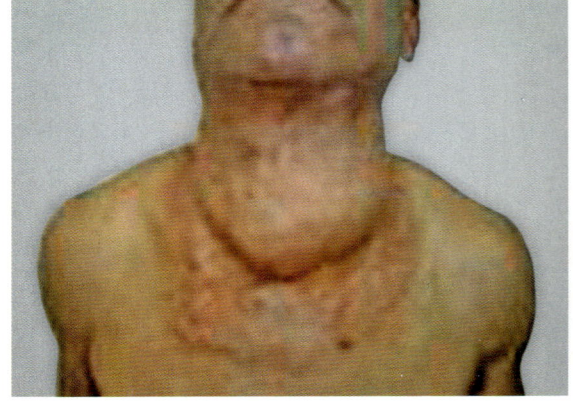

Fig. 30.8: Patient with thyroid growth

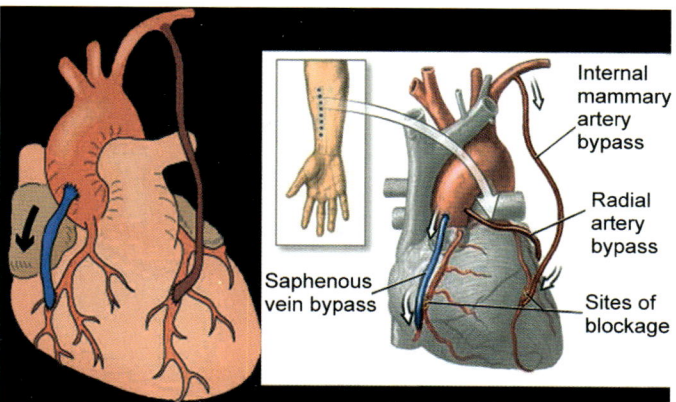

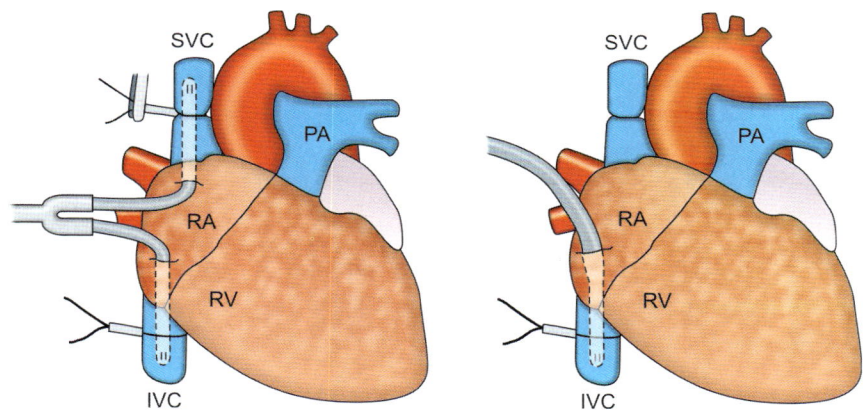

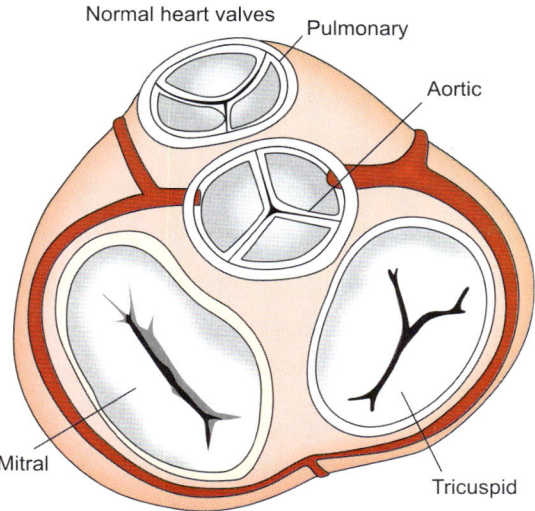

Fig. 30.9: Example of cardiac surgery and anatomy of heart

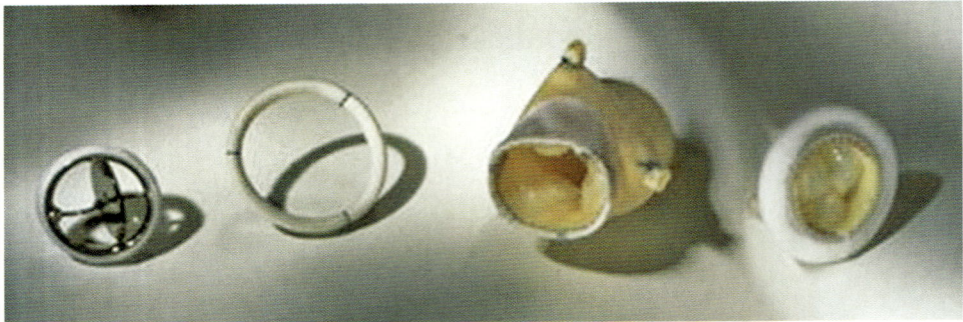

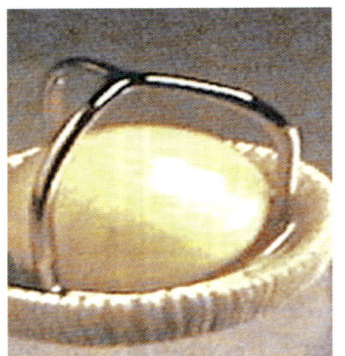
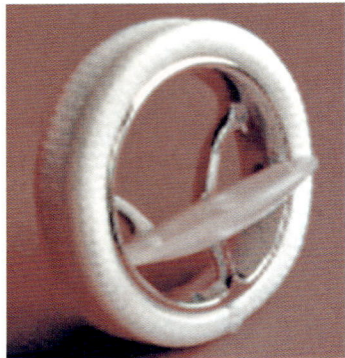
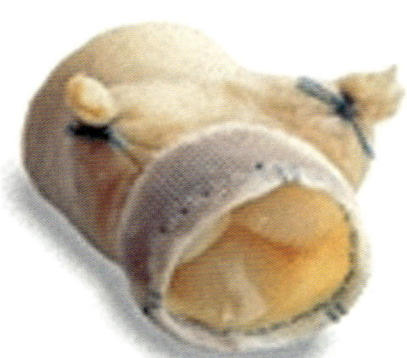

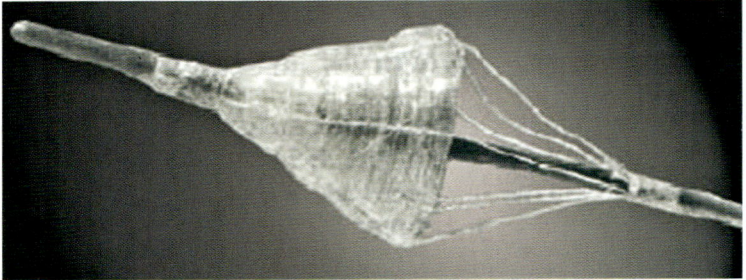

Fig. 30.10: Replacement of valve surgically implantation

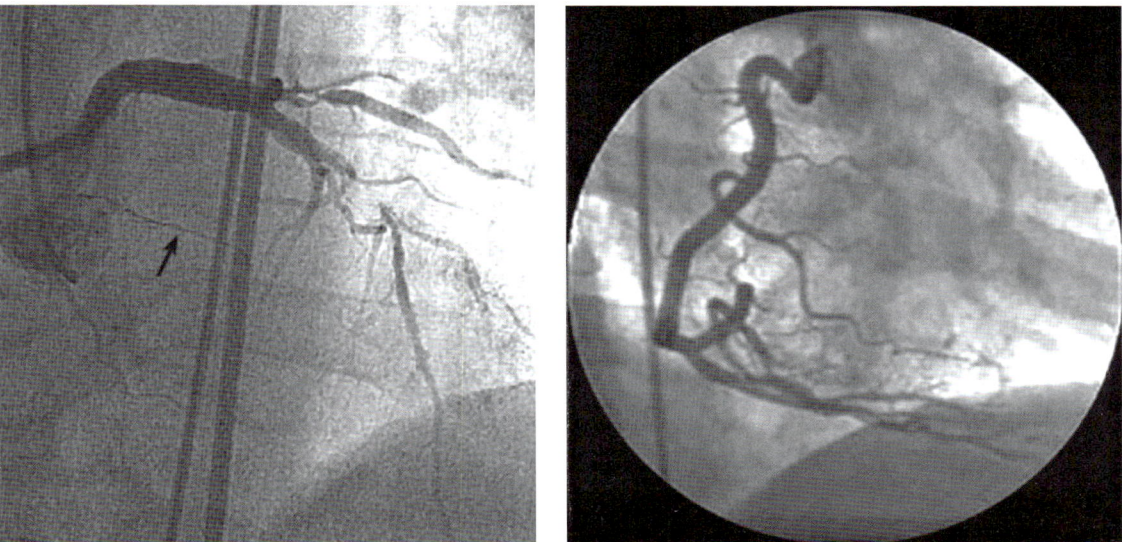

Fig. 30.11: Coronary angiography procedure

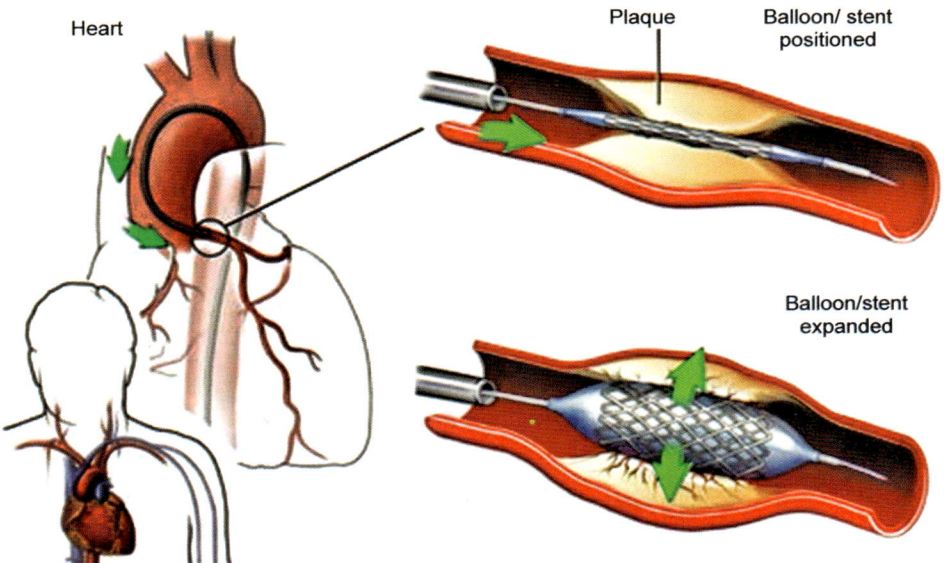

Fig. 30.12: Stenting insertion procedure

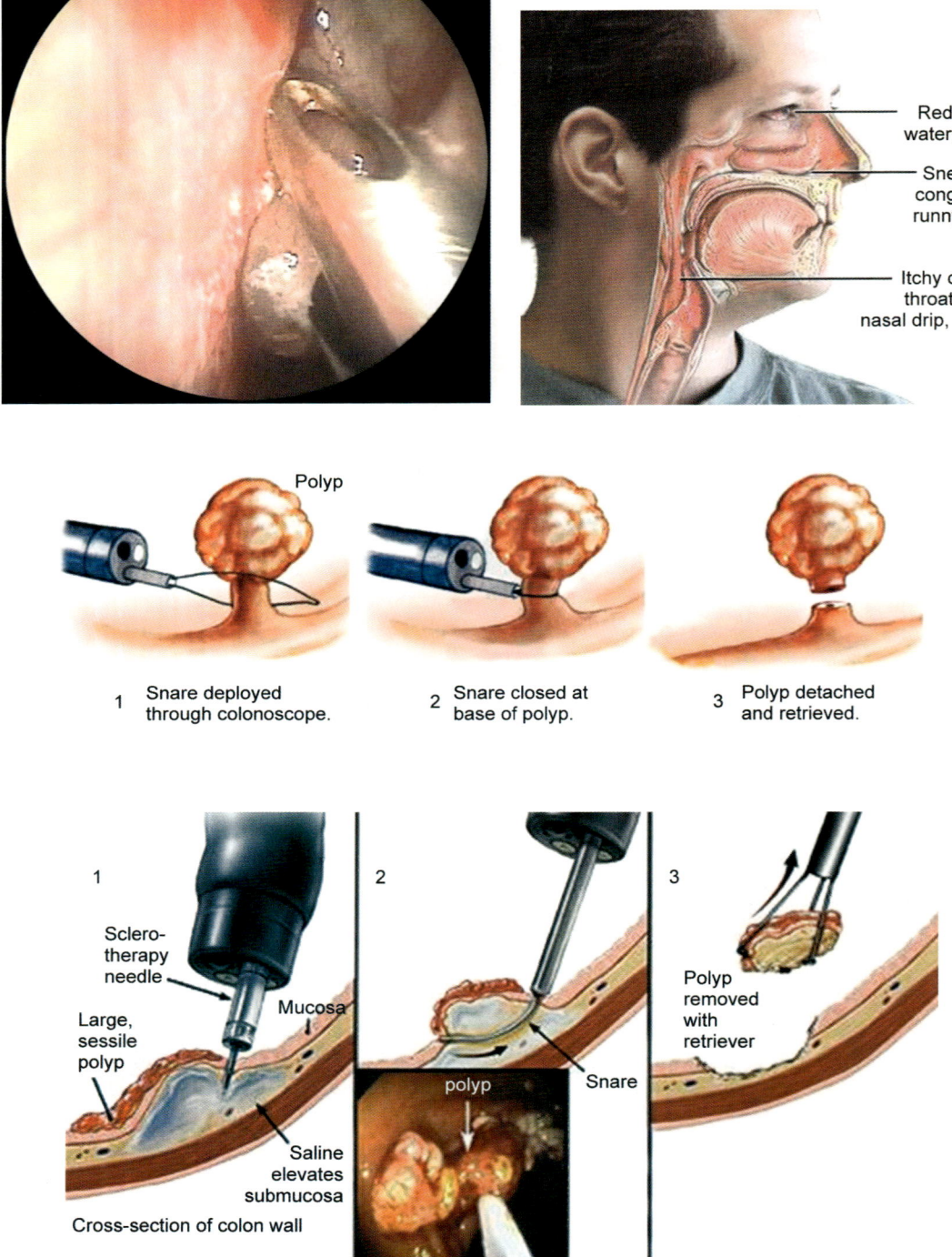

Fig. 30.13: Different site polyp polypectomy surgery

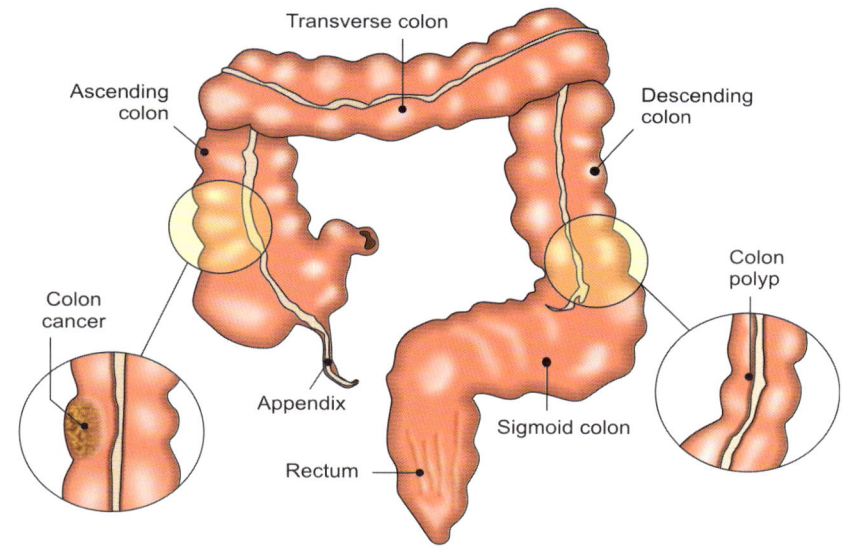

Transverse colon

Ascending colon

Descending colon

Colon polyp

Colon cancer

Appendix

Sigmoid colon

Rectum

Colon cancer and polyp

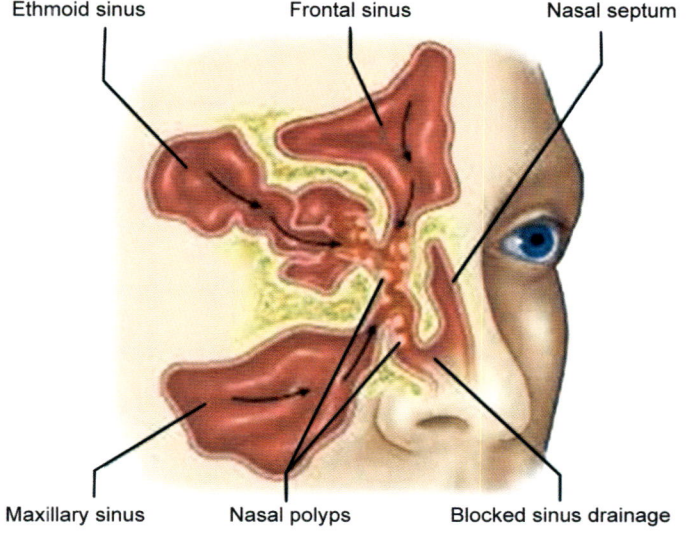

Ethmoid sinus

Frontal sinus

Nasal septum

Maxillary sinus

Nasal polyps

Blocked sinus drainage

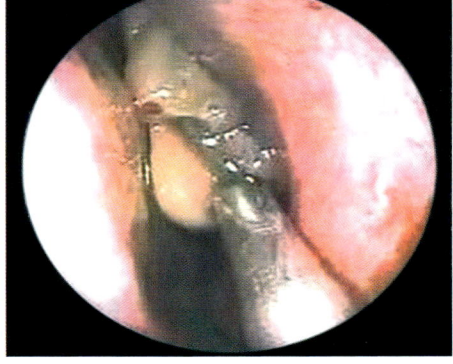

Fig. 30.14: Polypectomy surgery of colon

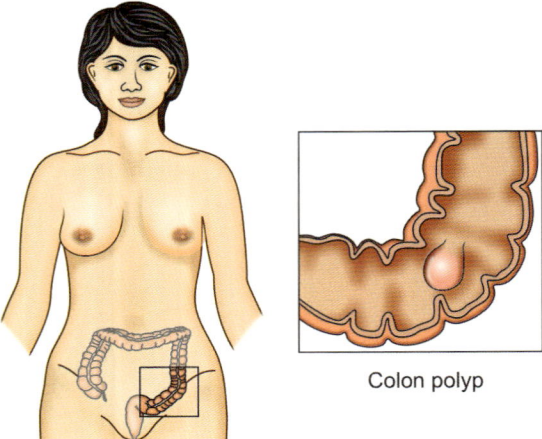

Colon polyp

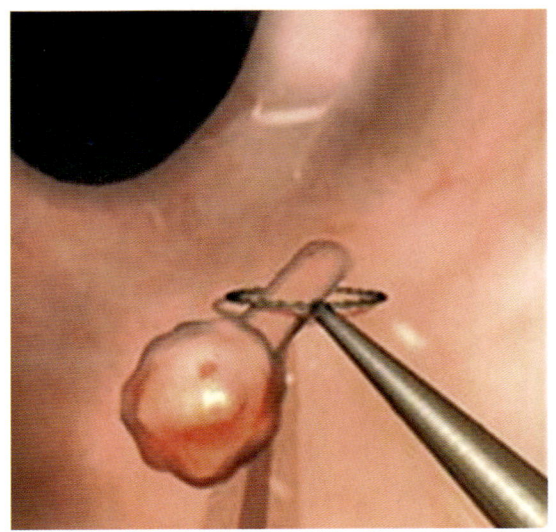

Turbinate-reduction

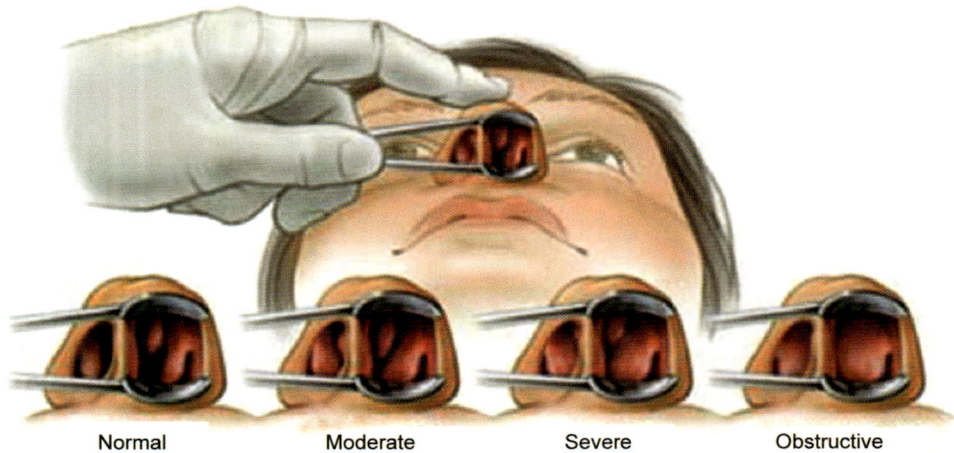

Normal   Moderate   Severe   Obstructive

Fig. 30.15: Polyp in different site surgically removed

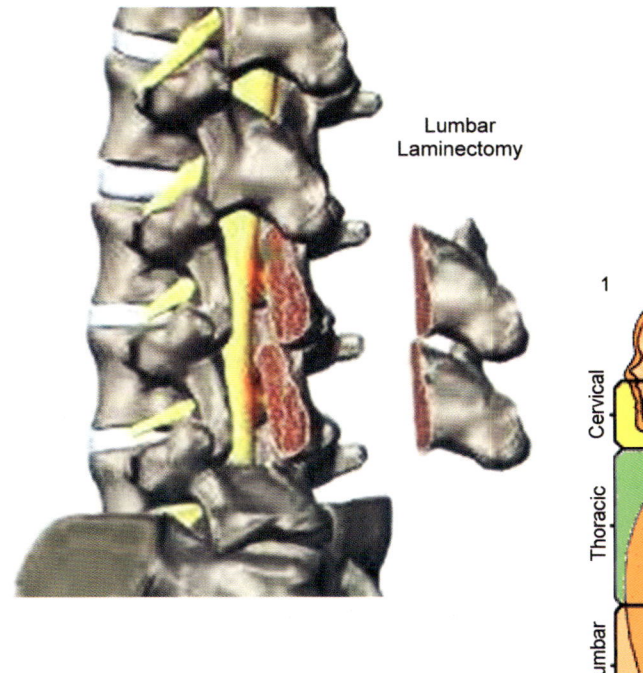

Lumbar
Laminectomy

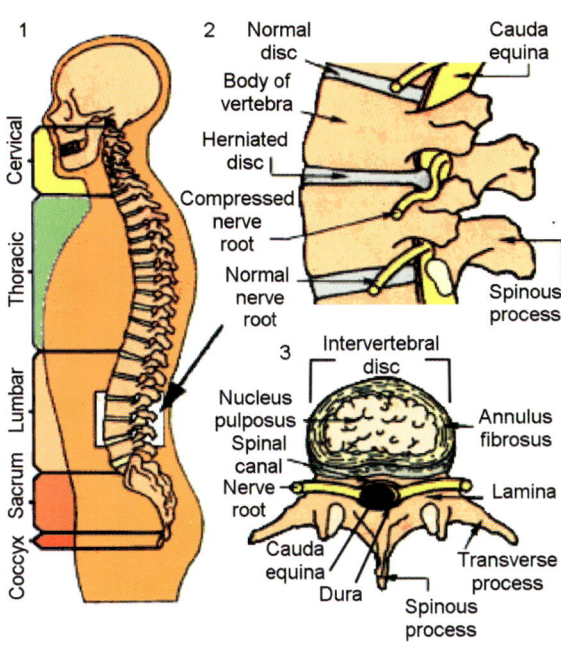

1   Cervical Thoracic Lumbar Sacrum Coccyx

2   Normal
     disc
     Body of
     vertebra
     Herniated
     disc
     Compressed
     nerve
     root
     Normal
     nerve
     root

Cauda
equina

Spinous
process

3   Intervertebral
     disc
     Nucleus
     pulposus
     Spinal
     canal
     Nerve
     root
     Cauda
     equina
          Dura

Annulus
fibrosus

Lamina

Transverse
process

Spinous
process

Laminectomy

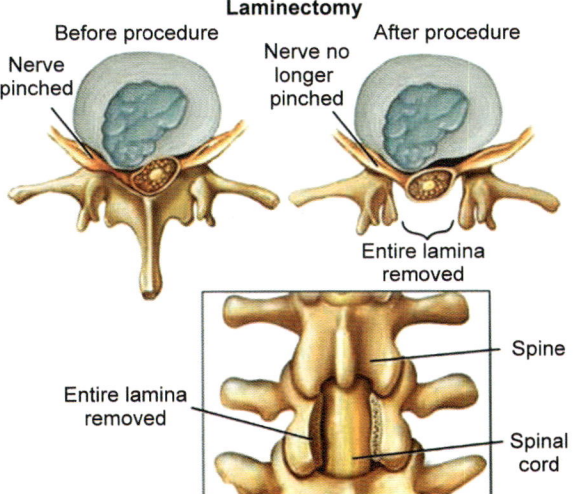

Before procedure

Nerve
pinched

Entire lamina
removed

After procedure

Nerve no
longer
pinched

Entire lamina
removed

Spine

Spinal
cord

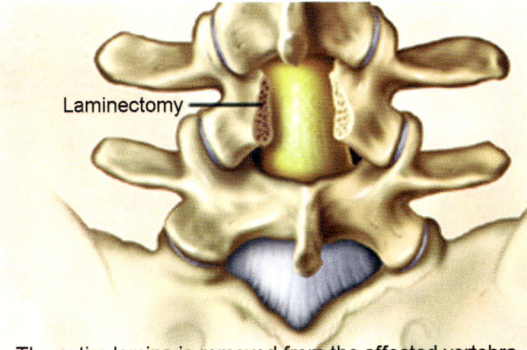

Laminectomy

The entire lamina is removed from the affected vertebra

Fig. 30.16: Laminectomy surgery

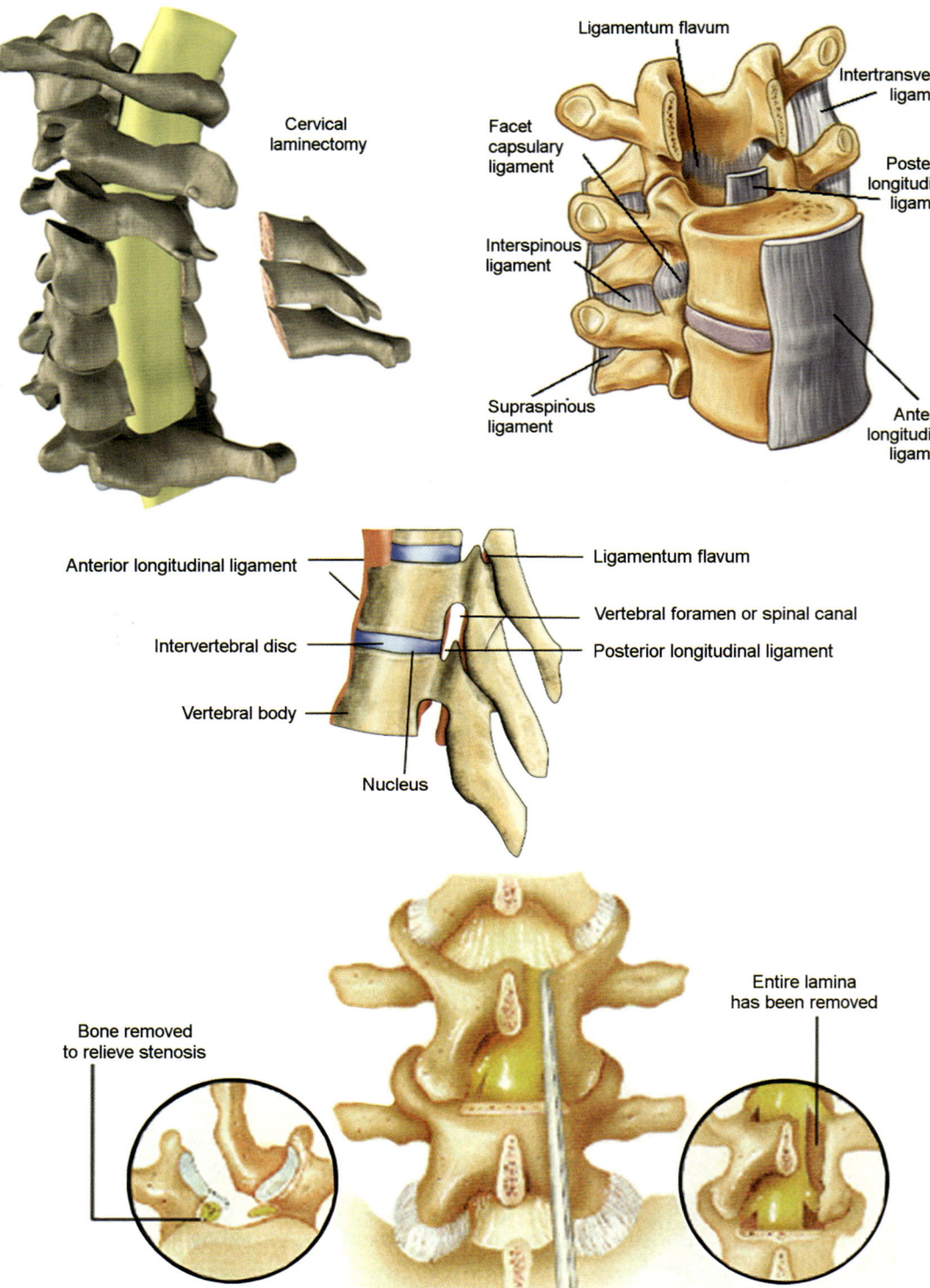

Cervical laminectomy

Ligamentum flavum

Intertransverse ligament

Facet capsulary ligament

Posterior longitudinal ligament

Interspinous ligament

Supraspinous ligament

Anterior longitudinal ligament

Anterior longitudinal ligament

Ligamentum flavum

Intervertebral disc

Vertebral foramen or spinal canal

Posterior longitudinal ligament

Vertebral body

Nucleus

Bone removed to relieve stenosis

Entire lamina has been removed

Fig. 30.17: Laminectomy surgery

4. Procedure is done by doctor using banding set
5. Nurse will assist the doctor
6. Resuscitation equipment and medications are kept ready
7. Monitor client during procedure
8. After procedure give comfortable position to client
9. Client is kept NBM after procedure for 1–2 hours after that for one day only liquid diet is advised and then soft diet.
10. Record and report clients condition in nurses notes
11. Recorded photographic reports are given to client
12. Explain for follow up consultation

Note: The above procedures are in figure form for the students to see and imagine the surgeries done in front of their eyes and widen there horizons into the world of surgery which is very vast in itself. It will give the nurse the interest and thirst for more knowledge that will vividly store into their memories for the years to come.

Index

Infections can spread 145
Infectious droplets 146
Information 62
Infusion 12
Inhibitors 26
Inserting 10
Interlock 88
Intermittent 17
Interpersonal 17
Intracatheter 25
Intradialytic 8, 25
Intraluminal 25
Intraoperative 76
Irreversible 57
Irrigation 101

Jaundice 33
Jugular 9

Kwashiorkor 45

Lacerations 28
Laryngoscope 127
Lifesaver 48
Loading 26
Lysoform 29

Maintenance 13
Malignant tumors 158
Mandatory 8
Manufactures 29
Marasmus 45
Mastectomy 93
Mastication 46
Matched 52
Medications 12
Membrane 9
Metabolism 43
Micro-organism 75
Milking 18
Misconception 52
Modifications 7
Molecular 28
Monitor 12
Monitoring 29
Mortality 37
Mutilating 47

Nasogastric 77
Nephrologists 8
Nephrons 55
Neurological 10
Neutralizes 26
Nocturia 56
Nonfunctional 25
Nursing is a service-oriented 152
Nutrients 45

Operation 14
Options for nursing 153

Organism to organ 160
Orientation 16
Osmosis 18
Osteoarthritis 54
Outlets 27
Oxidization 43
Oxygenation 75

Palliative 73
Parameters 12
Parameters 27
Pathology 58
Permanent 24
Placement of face mask 129
Platelets 28
Pleural fluid 123
Polycystic 48
Polytetrafluoroethylene 10
Posteriorly 83
Potassium 40
Povidone 24
Precautions 14
Prerequisite 9
Pressure 20
Principles 86
Process of globalization 153
Prolongation 26
Prophylactically 27
Prosthetic arms 155
Pseudoaneurysm 25
Psychological 14
Pump 11
Pyelogram 56

Quadriceps 96

Radiographic 109
Receptacle 10
Recipients 48
Recirculation 37
Reconstruct 51
Renaclean 187
Repositioning 25
Reprocessing 14
Responsibility 19
Restrictions 30
Resuscitation bag 127
Resuscitation equipment 183
Resuscitation 104
Retrieved 47
Roaster 17

Sagging 45
Sanitation procedures 145
Saturation 35
Schedule 15
Scissors 137
Screening 30
Scrubbing 77
Semipermeable 9

Septicemia 51
Serology 8
Sevoflurane 118
Simultaneously 35
Softener 23
Specimens 9
Splashing 28
Spontaneous respiration 129
Stabilize 24
Standards of cleanliness 147
Stenosis 25
Sterilization 91
Stock 17
Stretching 39
Subcutaneously 10
Suctioned 35
Supervision 13
Supplements 35
Surgical diathermy 137
Surgical needles 137
Surgically 9
Sutures 137
Synthetic 10

Tactile stimulation 129
Technicians 8
Termination 9
Therapeutic 7
Thrombolytics 25
Thrombophlebitis 78
Thromboplastin 26
Thrombosis 25
Tourniquet 19
Transducers 28
Transmembrane 18
Transmission 28
Transplantation 47
Trendelenburg 93

Ultrafiltration 9
Unacceptable 45
Unprecedented changes 161
Uridynamic 56
Urticaria 35

Vaccinations 13
Venous 24
Ventilator 53
Visualization 93
Vitamins 41
Volume 33

Ward housekeepers 148
Warmer 34
Waterproof 80
Withdrawal 34
Wristband 31

Xylocaine 64